WORK AND PLAY

RUDOLF ALLERS

WORK AND PLAY

COLLECTED PAPERS ON THE
PHILOSOPHY OF PSYCHOLOGY
(1938–1963)

Edited & with an Introduction by
Alexander Batthyany, Jorge Olaechea Catter,
& Andrew Tallon

MARQUETTE
UNIVERSITY
PRESS

MARQUETTE STUDIES IN PHILOSOPHY
NO. 64
ANDREW TALLON, SERIES EDITOR

www.marquette.edu/mupress/

FOUNDED 1916

LIBRARY OF CONGRESS CATALOGING-IN-PUBLICATION DATA

Allers, Rudolf, 1883-1963.
[Selections. 2008]
Work and play : collected papers on the philosophy of psychology, 1939/1962 / Rudolf Allers ; edited & with an introduction by Alexander Batthyany, Jorge Olaechea Catter & Andrew Tallon.
p. cm. — (Marquette studies in philosophy ; no. 64)
Includes bibliographical references and index.
ISBN-13: 978-0-87462-762-6 (pbk. : alk. paper)
ISBN-10: 0-87462-762-1 (pbk. : alk. paper)
1. Psychology—Philosophy. 2. Psychiatry—Philosophy. I. Batthyany, Alexander. II. Olaechea Catter, Jorge, 1976- III. Tallon, Andrew, 1934- IV. Title.
BF38.A36 2008
150.1—dc22

2008041597

About the cover photo: Private astronomical observatory of Karoly Nagy at the town Bicske, Fejér county, Hungary, completed in 1848-49. Photograph by Mathilde Windisch-Graetz.

♾ The paper used in this publication meets the minimum requirements of the American National Standard for Information Sciences—Permanence of Paper for Printed Library Materials, ANSI Z39.48-1992.

Association of American University Presses

MARQUETTE UNIVERSITY PRESS
MILWAUKEE

The Association of Jesuit University Presses

CONTENTS

NOTES ON RUDOLF ALLERS AND HIS THOUGHT

BY

ALEXANDER BATTHYANY & JORGE OLAECHEA

1. FROM THE EARLY YEARS UNTIL THE FIRST WORLD WAR

Rudolf Allers was born in Vienna on January 13, 1883, of Jewish extraction, the son of a doctor, Mark Allers, and his wife, Augusta Grailich. He was baptized that same year in Vienna's *Votivkirche*. The young Allers received his primary education at home, and although he received instruction in Catholicism, he would later recognize that he did not develop a real faith from family (Hoehn, 1948). He instead cultivated a great interest for art, music, languages – at Aller's home German, English, and French were all spoken – and books.

After finishing his studies in a secondary school focused on humanities, in 1902, Allers began to study medicine, convinced "that medical science could represent for his spirit a wide path into the world of the human being, a precious key that would be able to open up the mysteries of human life introducing him into the sacred depths of the soul" (Titone, 1957, p. 21). Although it was possible to attend Sigmund Freud's lectures at the University of Vienna, psychoanalysis did not interest him until 1908, the year that he was named assistant to the Neural and Mental Illness Clinic of the German University in Prague (under the guidance of Arnold Pick). There he met Dr. Otto Pötzl, who introduced Allers to psychoanalytic thought, of which he would afterwards become an "enthusiastic follower" (Allers, 1922, p. 15). In 1909 he became a psychiatrist and was transferred to the Psychiatric Clinic of Munich. There he worked as an assistant to Emil Kraepelin, one of the founders of modern psychiatry.

A year prior to his transfer, in 1908, he married Carola Meitner, of a Jewish family, who was the sister of the noted scientist Lise Meitner. During his time in Munich Allers came into contact with the phenomenological circle of philosophers living there, especially with Max

Scheler and his anthropological theories, and so distanced himself at the same time from the ideas of psychoanalysis.

In 1913 Allers started the work that he would come to love most: teaching at the university, as a psychiatry instructor in the Medical School of the University of Munich. The First World War, however, interrupted his teaching and he was put to work as a surgeon at the front, which earned him distinction from the Red Cross. Allers produced his first book during this period, entitled *Über Schädelschüsse: Probleme der Klinik und der Fürsorge* (1916). In it Allers compiled his research of physical and psychological traumas suffered by soldiers afflicted by gunshot wounds during the war. The endeavour to find links between physiological and psychological problems is already visible in his early work. The time that he dedicated to his philosophical writings would be no less important, as he recalls: "During the war (1914-1918); and the long periods of relative inertia in the field hospital, I was persuaded that the Thomistic philosophy offered the most adequate basis for the development of an "anthropological philosophical" system as the foundation of a theory of the normal and abnormal psyche" (Titone, 1957, p. 27).

2. IN VIENNA FROM 1918-1938

With the peace of 1918 "Allers served in the Medical School of the University of Vienna, working first in the department of sense physiology and medical psychology and then (from 1927) in that of psychiatry. He was able to blend teaching with laboratory research and a private practice. It was always against his complex background of teaching-research-therapy that he viewed the several schools of psychiatry which acknowledged Vienna as their radiating center. He became increasingly aware that psychiatric interpretations and methods were raising very general questions about man, and that the positions to which they led were laden with philosophical and religious implications" (Collins, 1964, pp. 282-283).

The first subject that he examined in depth was psychoanalysis. On April 26, 1920, Rudolf Allers gave his noted report *Über Psychoanalyse* before the Applied Psychopathological and Psychological Association of Vienna. In attendance were such notables as Schilder, Pötzl, Neumann, Pappenheim, Roffenstein, Federn, Hitschmann, and Stransky, who were among the great thinkers of psychology and psychiatry at that time. His criticisms of psychoanalysis were deepened and expanded in one of his most important works, written in English in 1940 and entitled *The Successful Error. A Critical Study of Freudian Psychoanalysis.*

According to Allers, psychoanalysis rests upon a gross logical fallacy: "Psychoanalysis, in fact more than once, takes for granted what it claims to prove and surreptitiously introduces its preconceived ideas into its reasonings so as to give the impression that these ideas have resulted from facts and evident principles" (Allers, 1940, 33). This fallacy, called in the field of logic *petitio principii,* was seen by Allers in the underlying principles of psychoanalysis, in the ideas of "resistance" and "association," and in the way of interpreting the analyzed facts where "interpretation and fantastic speculation take the place of observation and experimental analysis" (Allers, 1940b, pp. 256-257).

Allers criticizes the basic position of Freud about man: "Psychoanalysis is a thoroughly materialistic conception. It stands and falls with materialism. Whosoever feels incapable of accepting the philosophy of materialism cannot but reject psychoanalysis. Because of its materialism, the philosophy of Freud and his school is, in what regards ethics, a simple hedonism. It is addicted to an extreme subjectivism which even blinds the eyes of the psychoanalyst to obvious objective facts and truths. Because of its subjectivism it is impersonalistic and ignores the essence of the human person" (Allers, 1940b, p. 255).

In the meantime, Allers had familiarized himself with the ideas of Alfred Adler, to which he refers in a letter: "The most attractive element of his psychology was, in my opinion, the accent given to "man in his integrity," considered in the wholeness of his relationships and in the finality of human life, and as a consequence, his tendency of coping with behavior – even sexual behavior – as the expression of the fundamental tendencies of personality" (Titone, 1957, p. 27). Allers then entered into the Society for Individual Psychology, which he would later leave, in 1927. Within the Society he established, together with Karl Novotny, a medical work group that they would call *Arbeitsgemeinschaft Ärzte* (Lévy, 2002, p. 27). He also came into contact with Oswald Schwarz, one of the pioneers of psychosomatic medicine, notably contributing to volume edited by Schwarz on *Psychogenesis and Psychotherapy of Bodily Symptoms* (Vienna, 1925). That same year the young Frankl would collaborate with Allers in his laboratory work on the physiology of the senses.

The agreement with Adler's views, however, would not last very long. After becoming a psychiatry tutor, Allers decided to present his differences with Adlerian psychology more explicitly which led to his and Schwarz's exclusion from the Adlerian Society for Individual Psychology in 1927.

In the following years, most of which were spent in Vienna, Allers dedicated himself – alongside his teaching and research – to publishing numerous works, including some of his fundamental works.

The first and most voluminous work, *Das Werden der sittlichen Person: Wesen und Erziehung des Charakters* (1929a), written mainly for practical use (as pointed out by Allers in his introduction to the Italian edition), grounds his psychological practice on a study of the nature and genesis of human character.[1]

For Allers, character is something fundamentally variable, not simple nor unchangeable. This is the premise, according to him, for a theory of education that attempts to go beyond the mere transmission of content, or the training of a single faculty, in the individual. The concrete application of this type of character formation constitutes the content of the remaining chapters of this work.

In Allers' work, the attempt to rethink psychology and its applications based on a Christian view of man is already consistently present. It is interesting in this sense, to return to his concluding words: "We believe that we have made it quite clear that it was not our intention in this book to explain all the problems of character-formation and training with the help of recent advances of psychology, and that it cannot be maintained that the supernatural element can be excluded. On the contrary, we think that we have demonstrated *the limitations of natural means*; and we maintain that a purely naturalistic psychology, however complete and however well founded, must eventually break down unless it be co-ordinated with religious knowledge and principles. We have seen how problems arising of purely practical psychology and characterology immediately open up universal problems, insoluble except in terms of metaphysics, and that these problems lead us still further into the realm of revealed religion. Without being obliged in any way to involve ourselves speculatively in these ultimate problems, we are continually and inevitably being brought up against them" (Allers, 1931b, p. 375).

1 Allers had already dealt with the theme of character in some previous contributions (1924, 1929b).

During the following years Allers published many works: *Christus und der Arzt* (1931a), *The New Psychologies* (1932), *Sexual-Pädogogik. Grundlagen und Grundlinien* (1934), *Heilerziehung bei Abwegigkeit des Charakters: Einführung, Grundlagen, Probleme und Methoden* (1935a), *Temperament und Charakter: Fragen der Selbsterziehung* (1935b).

In these works Allers develops and consolidates his previous ideas on character and the human psyche in general, on psychology and its therapeutic applications. These ideas further clarify the interests that occupied Allers' future research, together with his interest in philosophical themes that are the foundation of an authentic vision of man. One of the first pages of *The New Psychologies* reveals Allers' awareness of this point: "The renaissance of metaphysics in our time shows a very characteristic feature: the first and most vivid interest centers on the problem of man; the most intensive search is for an anthropology. The great importance attached nowadays to all psychological questions is one example of this search. Today men have to answer this one question, put perhaps more earnestly now than ever before: What is Man?" (Allers, 1932, p. xviii).

Moved by this interest in philosophy, Allers accepted the invitation of Father Agostino Gemelli to pursue a doctorate in philosophy at the *Università Cattolica di Milano,* which he received in 1934. "His 'return to school' – says Collins – enabled him not only to deepen his acquaintance with the Greek and modern philosophical treatments of man but also to increase his intense interest in what the medievals had to say about man and his functions in the universe" (Collins, 1964, p. 283).

In the meantime, some important people had coincidentally visited Allers in Vienna. Hans Urs von Balthasar stayed at Allers' home for many months while he pursued his studies in German. Edith Stein lived for some time in the company of Rudolf, his wife Carol, and his son Ulrich (born in 1920), during her stay in Vienna in 1931. As Allers recalls in a letter to Hilda Graef, biographer of the German philosopher-saint, Edith spent most of the time at his home with them. Together they shared many interests and explored the following issues: the interest in philosophy and education of the person, the desire to articulate the best of mediaeval philosophical tradition with the developments of contemporary philosophy, and the problem of how to translate Saint Thomas into German in a way that would be both clear and faithful to the original.[2]

Another visit, probably in 1935, would be of great relevance for Allers' future. The doctor and psychiatrist, Francis Braceland, was struck by Allers' psychological works which were at that time circulating in English. After taking notice of Allers, Braceland was impressed also "by his broad humanistic grasp of history and languages, mathematics and music" (Collins, 1964, p. 284). He would be greatly responsible for Allers' move with his family to Washington, when the political situation in Nazi Germany became unbearable for them. So during the summer of 1937, Allers received an invitation by Father Ignatius Smith, O.P., dean of the School of Philosophy at the Catholic University of America, to become a professor at this important institution. Moving to Washington in 1938, he began to teach psychology to philosophy students.

3. FROM THE CATHOLIC UNIVERSITY OF AMERICA TO GEORGETOWN UNIVERSITY

There Allers began a new stage in his life. As a professor at the Catholic University of America, Allers immediately encountered the world of Catholic philosophy, at that time in full bloom in the United States. As early as 1938 he presented a report to the American Catholic Philosophical Association Congress on the concept of cause in psychology.

It would be impossible, in these few pages to attempt a summary of Allers' contributions during these years, ranging from psychological questions regarding legislation and marriage counselling, interesting analyses on the philosophy of mind, to historical studies such as his famous article (of almost 100 pages) *Microcosmus: From Anaximandros to Paracelsus*, for the journal *Traditio*. In addition to publishing the above-mentioned book on Freud and Psychoanalysis, during his first decade in Washington, Allers would publish only two other works: *Self Improvement* (1939) and *Character Education in Adolescence* (1940a). The rest of his publications are found in journals to which he regularly contributed.

2 Allers would translate into German Saint Thomas' *De ente et essentia* (1936) and Saint Anselm's *Monologion* and *Proslogion* (1936). In 1946 he would produce a translation into English of a text by Edith Stein: *Wege der Gotteserkenntnis: Die "symbolische Theologie" des Areopagiten und ihre sachlichen Voraussetzung* (1946).

Self Improvement is presented as an eminently practical work in which Allers attempts to show "that much more of the difficulties and troubles man has to wrestle with spring from his own personality" (Allers, 1939, p. v). It isn't a simple "self help manual," but a true phenomenology of certain problems that Allers considered should be understood by anyone looking for personal growth. A paragraph of the preface reveals the basis for the work: "This book is based on Christian philosophy and Christian morals. They supply the general trend of the reasonings, but they are not the point from which these reasonings start. All that is explained in the following chapters is based on experience. It is fact and not speculation" (Allers, 1939, p. v).

Practical value and concrete experience are not contradicted by assuming a particular position on man. The two perspectives must always go together. This cardinal idea in Allers' thought (that can be traced back to his earliest work) represents a fundamental intuition that must be reclaimed by today's psychology. The research into an adequate view of the human person is now more than ever imperative in the field of the psychological sciences.

Character Education in Adolescence is the collection of a series of articles by Allers in *The Homiletic and Pastoral Review*. It is an interesting contribution to the education of adolescents, who are the focus of his more outstanding psychological tracts. Again Allers' usual motive for using the concrete experience of adolescent males, which must be articulated in anthropological terms, is to provide an education that aims at their healthy development. Here a few selections offer a summary of the ideas of his work:

> Every practical measure, then, is determined by the ends which it is applied to realize. Educational measures, in particular, depend on what is believed to be the true aim of education. Science is absolutely and essentially incapable of discovering anything about aims. If someone tells us that we have to pursue this or that aim because of some statements of science, we may be sure beforehand that he is wrong; he may, of course, be right in recommending certain aims, but he is right, not because of his appeal to science, but in spite of it (Allers, 1940a, pp. 5-6).
>
> One may, of course, develop a certain technique of education; many things pertaining to education may be learned and taught. But the essence of pedagogy is nothing one can learn by attending lectures, nothing that can be fully explained in textbooks. Educa-

> tional influence is based on the personal relation between the educator and the educated (Allers, 1940a, p. 178).

Allers was sincerely appreciated by his students at the Catholic University of America. We have the testimony of James Collins, Allers' pupil from 1941 to 1944, in his article for the journal *The New Scholasticism* after the death of his teacher:

> Due to a highly developed memory and a delicate sense of proportion, Allers was able to present his materials in a steady thematic development without relying upon written notes, even when he made verbatim quotations from the sources. He gave one the impression of being totally and passionately involved in the topic under discussion, which he examined in an orderly fashion and yet with a sustained intellectual enthusiasm that was highly infectious among his students. They felt a special demanding quality about his lectures, which asked more rather than less of them if they were to appreciate what was going on. Allers did not have to preach about the integration of disciplines in the liberative mind, since his own example was there to observe and profit by. The act of teaching was for him a way of achieving, and encouraging others to achieve, a pertinent unification of the scientific and humanistic, historical and reflective, modes of human experience. The practical-exemplar character of this way of teaching was all the more effective for the fact that it never became divorced from the actual treatment of the problems at hand (Collins, 1964, p. 288).

In 1948, after 10 years of teaching, Allers was invited to Georgetown University by the then dean of the School of Philosophy, Father Hunter Guthrie, SJ, noted for having turned the faculty into a catholic think tank of great relevance by profiting from the contributions of European immigrants, including Allers.

There he taught philosophical anthropology. These would be years of intense study as he went into this field in depth. In his early 50s Allers would write: "I haven't yet written what I would desire to, that is, a comprehensive (integral) philosophy of human nature" (Titone, 1957, p. 27). And he never did it systematically. The classes at the university, however, offered him the space to develop his ideas.

As Collins points out, "it was during the Georgetown years, also, that Allers was able to bring to focus his lifelong concern with phenomenology and existentialism, especially as related to psychiatry" (Collins, 1964, p. 286). This interest would bear fruit in the volume

Existentialism and Psychiatry: Four Lectures (1961), a collection of lectures Allers gave at the Institute of Living (Hartford) where Braceland was director.

In 1957 Allers became Professor Emeritus, although he did not leave teaching until the end of his life. In 1952 his wife Carol had died. Three years after that Allers returned to Europe as a Fulbright Lecturer, giving conferences at the Universities of Paris, Toulouse, Vienna, and Geneva.

4. ALLERS' LAST YEARS

Allers' last years would be ones of distinction for the Austrian professor of almost eighty. In 1959 he gave the presidential speech at the Metaphysical Society of America on the question of the objective and the subjective (Allers, 1958/1959). In 1960 he received The Cardinal Spellman–Aquinas Medal from the American Catholic Philosophical Association. In that same year Georgetown University conferred upon him the honorary LL.D. degree.

After his retirement, Allers gave his lectures, first in the home of his son Ulrich (in Falls Church), and then in Carroll Manor, a nursing home in Hyattsville, where he spent time recovering from heart problems and from arthritis that weakened his health. As a note from a journal referred to him, "his students were brought by bus to Carroll Manor, where he taught in a solarium that the Carmelite sisters had made into a classroom." "Even in his later years when increasing disability limited him to a wheelchair, he continued to teach and his mind remained exceptionally keen," recorded *Ye Domesday Book* of Georgetown University.

From 1960 to 1963 Allers dedicated himself further to writing his last book, *Abnorme Welten*. In it Allers develops his knowledge of psychology and psychiatry, in an attempt to describe the "world" of those afflicted by these disturbances, helping create a new key for psychotherapy and psychiatric treatment.

Allers died December 14, 1963 from pneumonia.

The rediscovery of Allers' work can be enormously valuable to the study and application of the field of psychology. It is hoped that this brief work can serve to attract attention to this great thinker, who is undoubtedly relevant on account of the range and implications of his propositions, but who is nonetheless today "inexplicably forgotten" (Figari, 2005).

When the young Frankl prepared his first work on philosophy and psychotherapy – a work that should have been published by the Hirzel Press in the 20s – Oswald Schwarz wrote in the preface that this work would represent for psychotherapy what Kant's *Critique of Pure Reason* represented for philosophy: a radically new turn. Many years later, in 1958, Frankl affirmed in a letter to Oliver Brachfeld that on his advice, and "with more mature criteria," this phrase should be applied to Rudolf Allers (Brachfeld, 1958, p. 2).

BIBLIOGRAPHY

Allers R. (1916), *Über Schädelschüsse: Probleme der Klinik und der Fürsorge*, Berlin, Springer.

———. (1922), *Über Psychoanalyse: Einleitender Vortrag mit daranschliessender Aussprache im Verein für angewandte Psychopathologie und Psychologie in Wien*, Berlin, S. Karger.

———. (1924), *Charakter als Ausdruck. Ein Versuch über psychoanalytische und individualpsychologische Charakterologie*. In E. Utitz (*a cura di*), *Jahrbuch der Charakterologie*, vol. I, Berlin, Pan Verlag Rolf Heise, pp. 1-39.

———. (1929a), *Das Werden der sittlichen Person: Wesen und Erziehung des Charakters*, Freiburg, Herder.

———. (1929b), *Wille und Erkenntnis in der Entwicklung und Beeinflussung des Charakter*. In W. Eliasberg (*a cura di*), *Bericht über den III. Allgemeinen ärztlichen Kongress für Psychotherapie in Baden-Baden, 20.-22. April 1928*, Leipzig , S. Hirzel, pp. 113-124.

———. (1931a), *Christus und der Arzt*, Augsburg, Haas und Grabherr.

———. (1931b), *The Psychology of Character*, London, Sheed & Ward

———. (1932), *The New Psychologies*, London, Sheed & Ward.

———. (1934), *Sexual-Pädagogik: Grundlagen und Grundlinien*, Salzburg-Leipzig, Pustet.

———. (1935a), *Heilerziehung bei Abwegigkeit des Charakters: Einführung, Grundlagen, Probleme und Methoden*, Einsiedeln-Köln, Benziger.

———. (1935b), *Temperament und Charakter. Fragen der Selbsterziehung*, München, Ars Sacra Josef Müller.

———. (1939), *Self Improvement*, London, Burns Oates & Washbourne.

———. (1940a), *Character Education in Adolescence*, New York, Wagner.

———. (1940b), *The Successful Error: A Critical Study of Freudian Psychoanalysis*, New York, Sheed & Ward.

———. (1944), *Microcosmus: From Anaximandros to Paracelsus*, *Traditio*, vol. 2, pp. 319-407.

———. (1958/1959), "The Subjective and the Objective," *The Review of Metaphysics*, vol. 12, pp. 503-520.

———. (1961a), *Existentialism and Psychiatry: Four Lectures*, Springfield, Charles C. Thomas.

Anselm von Canterbury (1936), *Leben, Werke und Lehre*, Hegner, Wien 1936.

Brachfeld O. (1958), "Rudolf Allers, la 'Tercera Escuela Vienesa' y la pedagogía sexual." In R. Allers, *Pedagogía sexual y relaciones humanas: Fundamentos y líneas principales analítico-existenciales*, *a cura di* O. Brachfeld, Barcelona, Luis Miracle, pp. 9-48.

Collins J. (1964), "The Work of Rudolf Allers," *The New Scholasticism*, vol. 38, pp. 281-309.

Figari L.F. (2005), *An Inexplicably Forgotten Thinker: The Reappearance of Dr. Allers*, "Rudolf Allers Information Page" (http://www.rudolfallers.info/figari.html).

Frankl, V.E. (2000), *Recollections*. New York: Perseus

Hoehn M. (1948), *Rudolf Allers*. In Id. (*a cura di*), *Catholic Authors*, Newark, St. Mary's Abbey, pp. 6-7.

Lévy A. (2002), "Rudolf Allers – ein katholischer Individualpsychologe." In A. Lévy e G. Mackenthun (*a cura di*), *Gestalten um Alfred Adler: Pioniere der Individualpsychologie*, Würzburg, Königshausen & Neumann, pp. 27-36.

Sister Theresia Benedicta a Cruce (1946), "Ways to Know God: The 'Symbolic Theology' of Dionysius the Areopagite and its Factual Presuppositions," *The Thomist*, vol. 9, pp. 379-420.

Thomas von Aquin (1936), *Über das Sein und das Wesen: De ente et essentia*. Deutsch-lateinische Ausgabe. Übersetzt und Erläutert, Hegner, Wien 1936.

Titone R. (1957), *Rudolf Allers, psicologo del carattere*, Brescia, La Scuola.

INTRODUCTION

BY

ALEXANDER BATTHYANY &
JORGE OLAECHEA CATTER

In this volume, fourteen papers written by Rudolf Allers are presented in chronological order. Allers' publication list includes over 600 scientific and philosophical papers and presentations; certainly then, this collection of the articles consists merely of snapshots which are set out to reintroduce Allers and his work to a wider readership. The papers presented here have been written between 1938 and 1963, and Allers developed important new ideas during these years; yet there is a common thread which runs through his entire work. The same goes for this book. Indeed, if this volume can be said to have any single thesis or argument, it is that the dialogue between psychiatry, philosophy, and theology is not a dialogue across borders, but a dialogue between and about human beings. Whether he addresses the human person from disciplines as different as neurology, psychiatry, psychology, philosophy, and theology, Allers begins and ends each of his discussions and reflection with the implicit – and often explicit – acknowledgement that there is something enigmatic about being a human person; an enigma which we can try to understand, but not one which we can solve easily. In other words, understanding human personhood is not something which any one single discipline can claim to be able to achieve: but each discipline might add some knowledge about certain aspects of the human person. Yet it can do so only if it is understood to be part of vaster project, namely, a truly interdisciplinary research project – and one which refrains from mistaking explaining for reducing. Allers' own work is exemplary in this regard, and arguably, for a long time, stood alone. Perhaps here lies one the reasons why it was so easily forgotten. For psychiatrists, his writings might have been too philosophical; for philosophers, too medical; and for theologians, too scientific.

Indeed, from the outset of his work as doctor and researcher, Allers had not only allowed a variety of methods to apply; rather he straightforwardly promoted them. His model views body, mind, and spirit in the human being as aspects of a unity, whose essences are to be differentiated qualitatively, in order to be able with a single method to appropriately describe or treat it. And Allers had also anticipated something here that decades later for the first time would find entrance into the scientific landscape: the trend towards varying methodologies reflects itself today in the increasing interdisciplinary interdependence of the empirical behavioral sciences. These days we hear calls, and calls for that matter from many factions within the field of scientific psychology, for a systematic focusing of the research activities of different subject disciplines. It remains to be seen whether these calls will be heard and what concrete form its realization will take. In any case, however, we can determine that the recognition that there is not one but rather numerous sciences of humanity, was already a fundamental creed of Allers' conceptualization of the human being.

We editors believe that current trends in the behavioral and cognitive sciences provide a good basis for reintroducing Allers' work to a wider readership. It not only provides us with a history of a discipline which is currently in the making – consciousness research; it also serves as an exemplar of how the project of a non-reductionist, yet scientifically informed, philosophy of personhood could and should look.

THE ARTICLES

1. The conference presentation *Cause in Psychology* can be considered Allers' self-introduction to Catholic American scholarship. Having arrived in the USA from Vienna at the end of 1937, he was invited to address the Annual Meeting of the American Catholic Philosophical Association taking place on December 1938 in Cincinnati (Ohio), under the effective presidency of Fr. Ignatius Smith, OP, who was also responsible for the arrival of Allers at the Catholic University of America.

The paper calls attention to the actual importance of the notion of causality, not only in psychology but also in general philosophy. In a time when this notion was being extensively criticized and denied, especially in the field of physics, but increasingly in other sciences and philosophy, Allers tried to justify its necessity for an empiric discipline as psychology.

In order to do this, the Austrian psychiatrist describes the specificity of psychological research, which deals with "mental facts," "The argument of the physicist – remarks Allers in his conference – is quite incapable of "dissolving" the notion of causality because there is at least one field of reality, viz., the field of mental facts, whose essential conditions do not allow for introducing the idea of statistical laws. Psychology thus supplies a strong, indeed I believe an unanswerable, argument against the idea that the notion of causality is based on a misconception of reality."

Moreover, the paper recalls the many facts and problems faced by the psychologist whose explanations do not only require a general notion of causality (usually identified with the classic "efficient cause"), but also of a precise determination of the four "classic" causes: material, efficient, final, and formal. Finally, Allers stresses the importance of the idea of *analogia entis* to understand this issue: "As soon as one becomes aware of the merely analogical meaning of cause in psychology, many difficulties disappear and many problems are revealed as artificial and as due to a mistaken philosophy."

2. In *Irresistible Impulses: A Question of Moral Psychology*, written for the 100th volume of *The Ecclesiastical Review* (1939), Allers discusses the alleged "irresistibility" of certain impulses in normal persons and the responsibility (or lack of it) following these actions.

This essay represents an interesting application of some general premises developed in different works by Allers around the mid 20s. He emphasizes, for example, that in order to form an opinion on the irresistibility of the impulses, "we have to consider not this impulse as such but the totality of the conditions, inner and outer, existing at the moment of action," because "a human action can be really understood only if it is viewed in its totality." Another premise of the analysis is the distinction between "the objective irresistibility of an impulse and the subjective conviction that such is the case."

Allers goes back to the origin of the widespread idea of irresistibility and finds the pervasive belief that there are forces that drive persons to immoral or antisocial behavior, forces that must be alien to human intellect and will: "To safeguard the nobility and absolute supremacy of human nature these forces have to be subjected to irresistibility. [...] Materialistic mechanism and moral determinism could never get hold of the modern mind, if the true notion of original sin – and, accordingly, of human nature – had not first been destroyed."

Arriving to a judgment on irresistibility is not as simple as is usually believed. The analysis has to consider several distinctions that Allers briefly describes: the strength of the situation may arise from the force of the impulse, or from the knowledge that by not giving way to it some intolerable phenomena will occur; the irresistibility may be attributed to the impulse itself (as in certain actions caused by passion), or to the craving for relief (as in many sexual acts); the impulse may arise so suddenly and with such a strength as not to allow for consciousness, or it can reach the point of irresistibility only after some yielding.

The Austrian psychiatrist concludes that, as there are no reliable objective criteria of irresistibility, there is no impulse which may be considered as irresistible in itself. All generalization must be strictly avoided in this issue: "The most important thing is that every case is to be considered as an altogether new problem. [...] We cannot know anything of the true nature of the allegedly irresistible impulse unless we know all we can find out about the total personality."

3. "A closer study of certain empirical data collected by the experimentalists on one hand and an analysis of the true meaning of the Scholastic conception" are the two tasks assumed by Allers on the third paper, *The "Vis Cogitativa" and Evaluation*, which deals with the relation of the *ratio particularis* (or *vis cogitativa*) and the awareness of values. The essay has two parts.

The first one presents certain aspects of the Scholastic approach to this human faculty: its proper object and functions, its relation to the rational will and the intellect, and the cooperation between sensitive and intellective faculties. Reference is made primarily to the work of Aquinas, recognizing however "that St. Thomas himself did not consider his system as complete and closed." Allers discusses also some assertions made by John of St. Thomas in his *Cursus Philosophicus* about the data allowing the *vis cogitativa* to become aware of axiological relations. Following the reasoning of the commentator – concludes the author – "one arrives, with a certain inevitability, at an objectivistic conception of values."

In the second part, Allers moves on to study whether or not the Scholastic notion of the *vis cogitativa* is in agreement with the findings of experimental psychology, and specifically with that of research on value-apprehension. Allers makes extensive use of the experimental work of W. Gruehn in his *Das Werterlebnis*, emphasizing his findings on what he calls the "act of appropriation" of the value.

The concluding paragraph of the essay is emblematic of Allers' view of philosophy, psychology and their interrelation, and it is also relevant within the scope of the present book: "The situations in present philosophy and in present psychology point in the same direction. The gap between these two endeavors of man for understanding reality and himself apparently may become less wide. [...] But no co-operation can ever be brought about as long as the philosopher ignores the doings of the psychologist, and the latter thinks unimportant what the former says."

4. In the next paper – published in 1942 by the Dominican review *The Thomist* – Allers continues the presentation of his research on the cogitative power, regarding, in this case, *The cognitive aspect of emotions*. Allers moves from what in traditional – ancient and medieval – psychology is considered an emotional state, and its relation with the "total situation of behavior" to modern theories: the James-Lange-Sergi theory; the ideas of Max Scheler and Alexius von Meinong on emotional states and the awareness of values; the works of Sören Kierkegaard on dread and despair; and those of Martin Heidegger emphasizing the difference between fear and dread, the ontological notion of the Naught and the awareness of human finitude and contingency.

At the end of this overview Allers recalls that "if it is true that emotional states have, whatever their role may be besides, the function of revealing to man, in a peculiar manner, something of his position in the order of being, his 'ontic status,' and, accordingly, of his nature, it would be exceedingly improbable that only the negative emotions, like dread or despair, should be gifted with such a power." Thus he develops an interesting phenomenological analysis of some "positive" emotions as love, wonder, compassion, and admiration, arriving to a first conclusion on their "cognitive aspect": the mere experiencing of emotions does not offer the mind any definite knowledge unless the awareness they supply be combined with reflection.

The next part of the essay deals with some characteristics of emotions as interpreted by different psychologists: their passivity as pure responses; their lack of a peculiarity founded on other mental phenomena, that is, to present to the reflecting mind various aspects or sides (emotions are, in this sense, "absolute"); their being modifications of the experience the ego has of itself.

At this point a main question is raised: is there any relation between the generally accepted interpretation of emotions and the conceptions submitted in the paper? "The answer," emphasizes the author, "depends on the idea one forms of the situations to which the organism, or rather the person [...] responds by an emotion. According to the thesis defended here, these situations must be of such a nature as to provoke a realization of the 'ontic status' of man in general and of the individual person in particular."

Allers then responds to some objections to his position, concluding that emotions are just the means (the *id quo*) for awareness of values. They don't apprehend the value side of being in themselves. This operation is done by the cogitative power; existing, nevertheless, "a mutual influence (flowing to and fro, so to speak) of emotions and the correlated movements of the sensitive appetites on one hand, and the performance of the *vis cogitativa* on the other."

5. *The Limitations of Medical Psychology* is the title of the fifth essay presented in this book. It was published during the Second World War (1942) in Fordham University's quarterly *Thought*." Although brief, this paper is a good summary of some ideas Allers had already presented in different works regarding "medical psychology." By this name the Austrian psychiatrist meant the modern psychological positions which stemmed from medicine (especially from psychiatry or neuropathology), such as, for example, Freudian psychoanalysis, Adler's individual psychology, or Jung's modification of psychoanalysis.

This paper denounces the "imperialism" of medical psychology, as long as it "attempts to impose its categories and ideas on other disciplines where they have no application." And this imposition is made, on the one hand, on some particular disciplines that actually have their own parameters and notions (such as art or poetry, social sciences or education), becoming distorted in the analysis of their objects by certain psychological pseudo-explanations; or also, on other hand, replacing ethics or anthropological philosophy in determining what is good or bad, right or wrong, or defining the aims of other human disciplines by the "explanation" of human nature.

Extreme subjectivism and the devaluation of reason, the confusion of "facts" with certain discoveries presented in the language of preconceived ideas, the tendency towards narrowing as far as possible the range of responsibility, these are some traits characterizing modern medical psychology, which is guilty of what Edmund Husserl called the fallacy of "psychologism."

"Our age," says Allers, and it seems that things have still not changed in this regard, "is obsessed by psychology," and the reason for this phenomenon is that "recent times have lost the true and comprehensive conception of man's nature." Thus the importance given by the author to the re-construction and re-presentation of a comprehensive anthropological philosophy, on which he worked throughout all his life and teachings.

6. *Intuition and Abstraction* was born as an answer to remarks by Sebastian Day, OFM, in his work *Intuitive Cognition: A Key to the Significance of the Later Scholastics* (1947), where this Franciscan scholar refers critically to some articles of Allers. "However," states the Austrian psychiatrist, "I do not think that a purely polemic answer is very helpful; the idea to refute, if I am able to do so, point by point the statements of the author, does not appeal to me. [...] It seems to me that it would be better to raise some questions, to refer to some facts, and to draw certain conclusions independently of the reasoning so ably worked out by Dr. Day."

On which point does all of this controversy turn? The issue being debated is the intellectual cognition of particulars, and more precisely the existence or not of an *intellectual* capacity for *intuiting* particulars. In this paper, reference is made more to psychological experience and psychological facts than to Scholastic philosophy.

After a few words on some general problems concerning Day's approach to historical issues in philosophy, Allers focuses on the distinction between "knowing" and "knowing *about*," and presents the main thesis of his essay: "I shall try to show that it is not necessary for an explanation of certain intellectual performances to assume that the intellect knows particulars and knows them more or less in the same manner as the senses."

He analyzes sensory cognition, giving several arguments in favor of a theory that assumes some sort of mediation in this kind of knowledge as well. Bodily changes are the *medium* by which a particular material thing is known by our senses; they "mediate somehow between the *res extra* and our knowledge thereof." In a similar way – in intellectual knowledge – there is "something" that "mediates between the trans-subjective datum and the cognitive awareness thereof."

Allers has presented empirical data and has followed the difficulties that the theory of "intellectual intuition" encounters. From here he draws some conclusions: "the empirical evidence in favor of an intuitive knowledge of particulars on the part of the intellect is insufficient," "the reasons alleged for the necessity of such an intellectual intuitive knowledge are not cogent," and "the problems raised can be solved also on the basis of a theory which credits the intellect with abstractive knowledge only."

7. On September 1947, Rudolf Allers participated at the eighth symposium of the Conference on Science, Philosophy and Religion in their Relation to the Democratic Way of Life, a symposium dealing with "Learning and World Peace." Allers' conference – *Philosophia-Philanthropia* – assumed the task of inquiring "into the rational foundation of neighborly love, and hence of "'philanthropy.'"

First of all, he responds to a widely spread prejudice against philosophy, namely, that theoretical ideas have no influence on practical issues or in shaping man's life. Allers points out, rather, that "even if the real forces shaping man's life are other than that of reason, nonetheless these forces become effective mainly when they are formulated in an intelligible manner."

In this paper Allers emphasizes two characteristics of the development of "recent times." The first one is "depersonalization" (or "dehumanization"), that is, the growing presence of situations or forces that deprive man of his dignity; totalitarianism represents the most evident force insofar as it considers the person "as an instrument subservient to the State, the Party, or the Race." The second is "reductionism," a child of the negations of nineteenth century thought, an attitude that "destroys the manifold nature of reality," leveling down all that was considered "higher" in ancient times, especially some dimensions of human nature. Reductionism is particularly strong within ethical proposals as, for example, in modern utilitarianism.

What should be done? Which theoretical basis is likely to make "human" our living conditions and to stress neighborly love?

Allers indicates, as a primary condition for this "re-humanization," the recognition of human uniqueness. That means, on one hand, the uniqueness of human nature – the distinction between being human and having any other nature – and, on the other hand, the uniqueness of each human person, that one person is by no means interchangeable with another: "possessing dignity, a peculiar kind of worth or value, he becomes and only in virtue of this, the goal of the specifically personalistic attitude of love."

8. *Ethics and Anthropology* is the title of the paper read by Allers at the meeting of the District of Columbia/Maryland Conference of the American Catholic Philosophical Association, in December 1949.

To understand the proposition of this eighth essay, it helps to start from one of its conclusive statements, which can offer a synthesis of Allers' view of the correlation between these two disciplines: "A comprehensive, truly philosophical anthropology which would also render account of these facts – *salvare apparentia* – is still a desideratum. Without such a foundation, the science of ethics cannot either cope with the present situation or successfully answer to its critics. Man needs to understand himself again."

Allers describes ethics by emphasizing its "inbetweenness," that is to say its being placed "between" speculative philosophy on the one hand and empirical anthropology on the other. Because it is a practical discipline, ethics must apply the principles it expounds, considering "the factual situations in which men exist and the factors which determine or modify this application." Moreover, as a normative discipline, ethics "needs to know what are human nature and its abilities in general and how the latter are modified by personal or environmental conditions."

Besides these internal reasons for cooperation between ethics and anthropology, Allers stresses the importance of this relation in order to contrast the pervasive relativism of our time. He points out the philosophical roots – nominalism, idealism, positivism, pragmatism – of the contemporary relativistic attitude, remembering, however, that to these philosophies "is added the incapacity of modern mind to form an adequate notion of human nature.

As a consequence there follows the need for this tight cooperation and concern. Allers considers the two sides of it: it has a positive aspect, that is, the demonstration that a given kind of ethics is commensurate with human nature; it has also a negative aspect, which can be also called "apologetic," that is, the justification of ethics before anthropology. The main aspect, however, remains the positive aspect: to describe facts and show what human beings reveals about themselves.

9. In his paper "*The Dialectics of Freedom,*" a lecture held at the 1951 Conference on Science, Philosophy and Religion in their Relation to the Democratic Way of Life at Columbia University, Allers analyses the concept of freedom in view of its social limitations. To address freedom through the lens of its limits might at first sight appear to be a rather awkward way of looking at freedom, yet it is often implicitly held idea that freedom and authority are mutually exclusive, an idea that Allers takes to task. Allers argues that rather than being in opposition, freedom and authority depend on each other: without authority, that is, natural, value-based limits and guidelines, no freedom would exist. Nor is the concept of authority coherent without the basic premise that man could do otherwise, i.e., has the freedom to choose his course of action. Otherwise, the very concept of authority would be meaningless: authority exercised over persons who are not free would be no authority at all, but merely an affirmation or disapproval of what would have happened anyway. From the viewpoint of the person over whom authority is exercised, however, the important question is: towards which ends, and by which ways do I use my freedom; and how do I relate to authority? The latter question gives Allers the opportunity to point out that both terms are not only interrelated (in a dialectical relationship), but can be coherently held up under the premise of objective values. Otherwise, freedom and authority would cease to be interrelated, for both would mean nothing but mere arbitrariness, which, as Allers points out, undermines both freedom and authority. Indeed, authority ceases to oppose our freedom and offers us a chance to live up to the objectively valuable only if an objective order is recognized, because only then are we able to judge authority and only then are we capable of understanding the authority of values that direct us within our freedom. Allers closes this essay with an emphatic plea to apply these ideas and concepts to everyday life, and especially to political life:

> Two words ought to be written so that everyone may have them before his eyes. They should adorn the walls of our schools, and they should resound in the minds of every citizen:
>
> Democracy obliges.

10. Does a person's philosophy depend on the sort of person he or she is? This is the question Allers discusses in his paper "*Psychiatry and the Role of Personal Belief*" (1955). While Allers agrees that our traits and personality dispositions do indeed influence our world view, he strongly disagrees with the reductionism of world views which lies at the heart of the idea that a person's philosophy of life need not be judged in its own terms, for example, on its validity and coherence. In other words, Allers argues that one cannot bypass a person's rational or cognitive belief system by merely looking at the mainly unconscious mental processes. Thus, when it comes to the above question, it is, according to Allers, at least as justifiable to ask whether the sort of person one is does not also depend on the philosophy of life one has. When it comes to psychopathology, these questions of course become increasingly important: since a philosophy of life depicts reality to a person, it also offers it guidelines towards coming to terms and coping with that reality. Certainly, then, attitudes, convictions, and general conceptions of reality might predispose a person towards certain psychological disorders, or might influence the degree and form of certain already existing underlying disorders. Accordingly, there is a complex relationship between worldview and psychology – a relationship too complex to be solved, or rather dissolved, by a small set of premises which by way of simplification have to reduce one or more of the many factors at work. Allers here makes an important distinction between "case and person," a distinction so strong that he adds the word "versus" between the two. Any mechanistic account of the psychology of worldviews will miss the fact that a person's philosophy of life is an individual expression of his striving to understand himself and the world. No mere causative account will ever capture how a person navigates through the world, and once this fact is recognized, worldview and psychological processes start to become irreducible elements of one indivisible whole: Allers criticizes, for example, psychoanalysis and other mechanistic schools of psychology for missing this crucial point, for even if there were a complete causal (i.e., psychologically deterministic) theory of why a person adheres to a certain worldview, the worldview as such would not be acknowledged, let alone understood as a person's individual way to view himself and his place in the world. Finally, Allers takes a closer look at what he calls the "two ways open to man":

> When man realizes, not only theoretically but with the whole of his being, what his nature is – that of a finite being with infinite possibilities – there seem to be two ways open to him. One way is that of self aggrandizement, the insensate attempt to raise himself to the level of an absolute. He then falls into despair [...].
>
> The other way is that of faith. This is the way of Gabriel Marcel. But a faith that is capable of transforming man's being must be more than the acceptance of certain tenets and the fulfillment of certain obligations. It must become one with the person's being.

As to the role of personal belief, then, Allers argues that indeed worldviews do play an important role in the development and sustaining of mental disturbances, yet at the same time he points out that it is not the task of psychotherapy either to convert its patients or to indoctrinate them. But: "It is the task – and the glory – of psychotherapy to help a man caught in the meshes of neurosis, and thus deprived of the freedom to decide upon his own life, by showing him the way to arrive at a true picture of himself and his place in the order of being, of his task and his hope."

11. In 1960, Allers received the Thomas Aquinas Medal for his outstanding contributions to philosophy and psychology; he dedicated his address to the topic of *cooperation and communication*. Allers begins his talk by pointing out that the honour of a scholar lies not so much in who he is and his biography, but for what he has achieved as scholar and teacher. It is this separation which sets the scene of the ensuing discussion of the term communication and cooperation. For, according to Allers, both terms are the basic elements by which philosophy – indeed all sciences – can evolve and develop. Obviously, in everyday life, both communication and cooperation are important, but when it comes to our attempt to understand man and his place in the world, we follow in the footsteps of the great thinkers of the past, who communicate with us (through the works and ideas they left behind) as we cooperate with them (by understanding and expanding their works and ideas); the same holds true for us in relationship to future generations: we communicate not only with our contemporaries, but also with future generations by what we ourselves leave behind, and we cooperate with them by ensuring that the works of our predecessors remain available. Thus, whereas individual lives are transient, man's attempt to understand life and its laws, both philosophical and physical,

is a constant succession whose single elements are bound together by cooperation and communication.

12. In the next essay, "*Ontoanalysis: A New Trend in Psychiatry*," published 1961 in the Proceedings of the American Catholic Philosophical Association, Allers draws the American audience's attention to thinking about the continental branch of the existentialist psychiatry movement which started in Europe around 1930. The essay very much reflects the history of ideas in American psychiatry, where existentialist psychiatry arrived after a delay of more than 30 years; besides its historical setting, this essay contains an interesting and important in-depth analysis of the promises and pitfalls of bringing a decisive and explicit philosophical viewpoint into psychotherapeutic and psychiatric practice. Noting that the term "existentialist psychiatry" (or, as he prefers to call it: ontoanalysis) stands for a number of different school of thoughts, Allers maintains that the common denominator of these different branches is the acknowledgement of the uniqueness of the individual person. No matter how promising this program sounds, however, Allers points out that once philosophy and psychiatry focus on the individual rather than the disease, they are confronted with a severe methodological and epistemological problem – they attempt to address the individual human being and his personal life situation, his conduct, his biography, his strivings and yearnings, and yet, at the same time, they are trying to present general guidelines for understanding that same individual, thus sacrificing the idea of "individuality" at the very moment they attempt to convey general truths about individuals rather than about only one individual.

The problem unfolding in this context is as much methodological as it is epistemological and is, in the contemporary philosophy of mind, better known as the epistemic asymmetry between the perspectives of the first person and the third person, except that in this case, the problem of the relationship between objective and subjective description is also a matter of disorder and mental health.

Indeed, the existential schools of psychiatry face a dilemma many a psychiatrist faces once he or she tries to acknowledge, rather than merely diagnose, the subjective world of the patient. In its attempt to bridge the gap between individuality and generality, existentialist psychiatry argues for an expansion of our understanding of the patient and his subjective world. While Allers views this philosophical program as a welcome and necessary addition to psychiatry and psychotherapy, he takes to task a common misunderstanding of existential psychiatry, namely, the idea that the only alternative to the strict positivism and scientism of a psychiatry arising from pure third-person perspective is the dissolution of the gap between objectivity and subjectivity and with it, the giving-up of any hope for objective discussions of mental processes and subjective worlds. But, as Allers points out, "it should not be forgotten that one may make objectively valid statements on subjective data," A rational alternative – Allers only hints at this program in this short review article – would be to follow exactly what the metaphor of perspectivity implies: to understand that one's understanding is bound to remain limited if one exclusively reduces the human person and his or her world to one perspective (or denies any such perspectivity) instead of accepting the scope and limits of each path to the reality of patient, world, and therapist.

13. According to a well-known proverb, there is a time to play, and there is a time to work. But when it comes to finding a clear definition of what separates work from play, we are often at a loss. One might, for example, argue that work is serious whereas play is not, but as Allers rightly points out in the next article, "*Work and Play" (1962)*, children are often very serious when playing, and so are many adults, for example, when playing tennis or chess. Given the fact that it is not easy to clearly and unequivocally distinguish the two, a number of educators suggest that the distinction is more a question of semantics than of real difference. Yet it is exactly at this point where Allers expresses his strong disagreement. He especially takes to task a current trend in educational psychology which suggests that a child's introduction to work should be playful, a trend that tries to obliterate the difference between work and play. Of course, such a criticism first needs to be set against a workable background definition of work and play, which is why Allers dedicates the greater part of his essay to the defining criteria of work and play: work, according to Allers, is an activity which is directed towards an achievement beyond the activity of work as such (and thus is intentional), whereas play has only one achievement, namely pleasure. While work is aimed at the changing or advancing something, play is an end itself. Importantly, this difference also affects the emotional outcome of work: the gratification of work and the gratification of play are both goal-directed and state-directed:

work is a gratifying experience if accompanied by achievement and accomplishment, whereas play is a gratifying experience as such – it gives pleasure. Against this background, Allers argues that both activities are important parts of a person's life, provided that the distinction between the two is upheld and understood. Play enables children to discover their abilities and limits, but with maturity comes responsibility for the ends towards which people deploy their abilities. The blurring of the distinctions between play and work is therefore highly problematic since it does not acknowledge what distinguishes the latter from the former: the value-orientation, responsibility, and sincerity that mature persons have to bring to their work, no matter how playful they otherwise might be.

14. The last and shortest paper ("*The Freud Legend,*" published posthumously in 1964) stands out from the other, more philosophical papers collected in this volume by being mainly a psychological study that contributes to the history of ideas as well as to Sigmund Freud's biography. Allers, who once was a close follower of Sigmund Freud and an eye-witness of the history of the development of psychoanalysis in Austria (until 1937), shares his perspective on the early Freudian movement and finds a number of conscious or unconscious misrepresentations both in Sigmund Freud's own recollections as well as in the biographical works of his followers, and attempts to provide a corrective view of the history of early psychoanalysis; his study is an important historical testimony.

CAUSE IN PSYCHOLOGY

The notion of causality is much discussed since some time. This fact is well known and needs no further illustrations. Psychology, however, has but little contributed to these discussions, though psychology uses the notion of causality hardly less than do other sciences, and though there are several important problems which can not be studied unless the place held by causality in psychological theory is precisely defined.

Many of the statements on mental things – made by the layman or by the student of psychology – would have, indeed, to be restated and revised if the category of cause could be shown to be invalid or out of place in psychology. The doubts raised on behalf of the meaning of the term cause can not but interest every science using this category.

The general situation of psychology makes an inquiry into the principles of this science rather desirable. We all know that there is not simply psychology, but that there are many psychologies. The controversies between these schools are not on facts; they are on theories and, mostly, on the general idea of psychology itself. If a theory of psychology, a "*Wissenschaftslehre*," of this discipline could be worked out, there would be some hope of reaching an understanding at least on the basic principles. This task demands for a careful analysis of the notions which form, as it were, the framework of psychology. Cause is doubtless one of the most important.

A study of causality in psychology may, however, become important also for the theory of causality in general. Every psychologist and every philosopher, he may hold whatever an idea on the nature of mental phenomena, has to acknowledge that mental facts are essentially different from all other ones. Even the absolute idealist has to recognize that the datum, mental fact, is of another kind than the one, physical fact. As long as account is taken of the phenomena, nothing of which the mind is aware can be confused with the awareness of the thing. Nor can the materialist, though he considers mental phenomena as peculiar manifestations of physical processes, be ignorant of these peculiarities. He, indeed, fully recognizes the differences between the two sets of phenomena, since he feels the need of "explaining" the one by the other.

Mental facts constitute a field of reality which is characterized by features missing in other fields. If there is some truth in the statement of certain modern physicists and philosophers that the notion of cause has been "dissolved," then this notion must be meaningless also in psychology. If, however, psychology is able to prove that causality has to be retained as a basic category, the aforesaid statement of physics becomes doubtful, at least it loses he generality with which its defenders credit it.

The discussion on causality has, indeed, been started by the physicists. Some of them see reason not only for abandoning the notion of causality in their own field but for declaring it null and meaningless wherever it is used. In this the physicists doubtless went farther than they were entitled to go. Even if they were right in regard to the physical world, they can not hope to "dissolve" the notion of cause outside of physics. To prove that causality has no meaning and no place among the categories of scientific thought one would have to dethrone it everywhere, and not only in physics.

If the physicists and the philosophers siding with them were content with exiling the notion of causality from physics nobody would find fault with them. One might point out to them that they did but discover a fact which by conscientious analysis of their own science they might have discovered long ago. The fact that physics do not use nor need the notion of causality has not been revealed to the physicists by some latest discoveries but by the awakening of what one may call their epistemological conscience.

A long time ago the physicist Ernst Mach had demanded that the notion of causality ought to be discarded in physics and that it ought to be replaced by the one of mathematical function. Mach had recognized that the proper object of physics is quantity or the quantitative aspect of physical reality. Causality, however, names a relation between things and not one between quantities. It is a common but an unprecise way to describe facts by saying that, *e.g.*, the weight of a stone caused the window to be smashed; the cause is in truth the stone itself, surely by its weight, but not the weight as such. Causality does not come in in physics, because physics do not deal with the things. The logical conclusion is that physics is incapable of deciding anything on causality. Many physicists, however, apparently feel differently. They still believe that their science is the one which gets the mind in touch with reality and reveals the very nature of things. But the so-called "world-view" of physics is very incomplete and very unsatisfactory; it is, in truth, no view of the world, since it has to be content with making statements on but one side of reality. Human mind, when eager to know the truth on reality and trusting to the lead of science, soon becomes aware that the full meaning of reality cannot be attained by this means. Science is, indeed, what Theodore Hæring once aptly called it, a *"Resignationsstufe des Erkennens"*; it is not the fullest, but a rather poor idea of reality we get from science.

The conviction, however, that science is the very way to approach reality and that science alone is capable of telling us about reality made those who believed in this creed believe also that causality had no meaning, because it had no place within their system of categories. Instead of concluding that science gives but an incomplete picture of reality, they preferred to conclude that causality had no place in reality.

The rejection of causality as a category of reality rests, therefore, on a prejudice or on a mistaken idea of the place held by physics within the totality of knowledge. There is, however, a second reason alleged by modern physicists.

The brilliant researches on infra-atomic physics and on "micro-events" have culminated in the development of statistical physics and in the discovery of the famous "uncertainty-relation" of Heisenberg. No need of recapitulating here the facts. The general idea is that the laws established by "classical" physics on "macro-processes" are no laws in the strict sense of the term, but the expression of statistical averages, and that the infra-atomic processes do not obey any law at all. The notion of causality is thus replaced by the one of probability. The extension of the conclusions, drawn on behalf of causality, to extra-physical fields is based, of course, on the same mistaken idea on the rôle of physics which has been just mentioned. But there is another fallacy involved, too.

Let us, for sake of argument (*posito sed non concesso*), suppose that physical laws are indeed laws of statistics only and that the micro-processes are not subjected to any law whatever. Let us concede, too, provisionarily, that by this the validity of causality in physics is abolished. Even if these statements were absolutely convincing, they still would not prove anything in extraphysical fields unless it can be shown that the same conditions obtain there as they exist in physics.

The argument of the physicists rests on the supposition, or may be the fact, that all "macro-events" have to be interpreted as the result or the aggregate of an infinite number of "micro-events," The notions of average and of statistics have a meaning only when and where we may suppose such elements to exist thus that by their combination a complex phenomena may be brought about. The argument of the physicist, accordingly, loses its sense as soon as the concept of "elements" cannot be applied any more.

But this is just the case with mental phenomena. There are no "micro-phenomena," no elements which, by addition and combination, might build up the "macro-phenomena," Even if we were to return to the ill-fated and luckily almost forgotten ideas of sensistic psychology, and if we were to suppose that mental phenomena "consist" of sensations, the situation still would be quite different. Sensation itself is still a "macro-phenomenon," and it obeys definite laws. There is no possibility of subdividing sensation into still more simple elements. Sensation is, even to an atomistic psychology, an *ultimum datum*. The laws of sensation – to mention only these – cannot be considered as statistical laws. The facts and ideas on which the physicist bases his criticism of causality have no analogy in psychology.

From this an important conclusion may be drawn: the argument of the physicist is quite incapable of "dissolving" the notion of causality because there is at least one field of reality, *viz.*, the one of mental facts, whose essential conditions do not allow for introducing the idea of statistical laws. Psychology thus supplies a strong, indeed I believe an unanswerable, argument against the idea that the notion of causality is based on a misconception of reality. Whatever physics may do with causality, there is no reason for abandoning it. Psychology and philosophy of nature may go on using this indeed unavoidable notion. It is so unavoidable that even the physicist cannot help reintroducing it surreptitiously; it is, indeed, implied in such notions as average, statistics, and probability.

Psychology may proceed to study the problem of causality within its own field, untroubled by the presumption of the pseudo-philosophy many physicists and quite a few who call themselves philosophers indulge in today.

The student of psychology who, keen to know something on cause in psychology, turns to the textbooks and treatises is sure to be disappointed. He may peruse many of them without even coming across the question of causality. Most psychologists, of course, assume that there are causal relations in mental life, but they do not care to define them more precisely. They take the existence of these causal relations as granted; but they take as granted, too, that the notion of causality as used in psychology cannot but be exactly the same as used in physics. They feel no desire and no reason for inquiring into the nature of these causal relations.

This rather curious indifference in face of an after all important and central problem has several reasons. One is the way psychology developed during the XIXth century; physics were then believed to be the ideal of knowledge, and every science was considered the more scientific the more its categories and methods resembled those of physics. Philosophy had, furthermore, lost nearly all credit, and if it had not, it had forgotten the Aristotelian and Scholastic ideas on causality. Of all the various kinds of causality which the older philosophers took so much care to distinguish efficient causality alone was known. Even Brentano's *Psychology*, which first appeared in 1878, does not mention the problem of causality, though its author was fully acquainted with the philosophy of Aristotle and knew something of Scholastic philosophy, too.

There are certain eternal problems of philosophy which may, indeed, be neglected for some time, but which will turn up ever and ever again. Each age has to define its attitude against these problems according to its general mentality and its cultural peculiarities. Whenever the historical, political, philosophical situation becomes entangled in a "crisis," all the problems will reappear, even if they have been qualified as obsolete and as done with by the preceding generation. Causality is one of these everlasting problems.

But a short time ago the average scholar would have looked askance at everyone daring to mention the terms of final, of material, or of formal cause. Such words were to be found only in treatises on the history of philosophy. A great change has come over the philosophical world. One is allowed again to use those notions without being labeled as an obscurantist and as lacking modernity. Very "progressive" scholars will not shun any more introducing such terms. It is the same with other notions, too. The name of "mental faculty" used to be quoted only to make fun of and to wonder at the useless subtleties of untrained minds. There are today quite a few psychologists who either recognize the notion of mental faculty or who use it under another name and perhaps without being aware of the fact.

The necessity of introducing the four classical kinds of causality becomes nowhere more apparent than in psychology. A discussion of cause in psychology is indeed impossible unless all the four causes are considered. There are some problems which escape the attention of the psychologist who is not ready to accept the other forms of cause besides the one of efficient cause.

The points which are at issue when the question of cause is raised are of different kind and, as it were, of different dignity. They may be grouped under the following heads:

1. The causal relations of bodily states or changes and mental phenomena. Under this head we have to comprise the facts of sensation or perception and certain connections obtaining between bodily processes and emotional states.

The unsophisticated mind is sure that the affection of the sense-organs is the cause of sensation or of awareness of a sensible thing. We may as well put in here a remark of a more general signification on the rôle played in scientific psychology by the convictions of the naïve mind. The conviction mentioned and others of the same kind are in themselves mental facts of which psychology has to take notice. Every science has to start from the phenomena; the *salvare apparentia* is an unavoidable task of science, and its neglect becomes a very serious drawback of every science.

It is, therefore, a grave mistake to declare some naïve conviction – based as it is on an immediate awareness – as an illusion and to "explain it away" by some theory. A theory of this kind which gives not a satisfactory reason for the existence of such an "illusion" is useless. The theory of psycho-physical parallelism may, *e.g.*, appeal to many as a self-consistent and clever interpretation; but it fails absolutely in explaining the arising of the idea of interdependence of mental and bodily states. This idea, however, is not the result of speculation, but the expression of an immediate experience. As long as no satisfactory explanation of one of these so-called illusions has been devised, so long we are obliged to accept the fact as it appears.

The problem of causation of the mental states of sensible awareness does not exist for the materialist, because to him the mental states are but concomitant to changes in the brain-cells. But he will still have to give an account of how the processes going on in the brain come to be contents of consciousness. The problem remains, even for the materialist, essentially the same; it is only located elsewhere.

There are evidently instances of emotional states being caused by bodily changes. Theories like the one proposed by James and Lange have, indeed, to be abandoned; too many facts contradict these theories. But it is true that somatic processes like those which normally accompany some emotional state may cause the very state to arise. Anxiety, *e.g.*, is accompanied by certain circulatory and respiratory phenomena; troubles of the heart or the respiratory apparatus may cause anxiety.

2. Man has, on the other hand, the evidence of mental phenomena becoming the cause of bodily changes. This is the case with action, be it more automatic or instinctive, be it of the type of voluntary action. It is also the case with the "expression of the emotions."

The relation of will to action appears at first sight to be the very reverse of sensation. In sensation the bodily affection of the sense organ causes the mental phenomenon of awareness of sensible things; in voluntary action the will causes the bodily changes, movements and the correlated phenomena building up action. There is no doubt that the mental phenomenon of will is experienced as the proximate cause of action. But will itself is caused by something. It is incorrect to say that will is caused by the idea or the image of a future situation to be realized by action. What moves the will – if the principle of freedom is discarded for the present moment – is not the image of the thing, but the thing itself of which we have the image. This thing, however, is a future thing, one which does not as yet exist in reality; it can, therefore, not influence the mind in the manner of an efficient cause. In studying the phenomena of voluntary action we are led by the phenomena themselves to introduce the notion of final cause.

This fact has been overlooked by most of the psychologists, at least by those who belonged to a more naturalistic and anti-philosophical school. But a conscientious analysis of the phenomenon reveals doubtless the fact mentioned before: we are not moved by images, but by the things of which these images are. We are also not aware of images in perception, but of things. The newer development of psychology, or of some schools of psychology, has tended towards a greater exactitude of observation of simple facts. The influence of Brentano and, more so, of his pupils, like K. Stumpf, E. Husserl, A. von Meinong, has worked towards sharpening the empirical conscience. Psychology has learned to distinguish the object from the content by which it is presented to consciousness, and both from the "act," which, indeed, is nothing else but the actual operation of the faculty.

The bodily phenomena accompanying emotions are felt to be caused by the mental states. Everyone is sure that he is trembling because he fears a danger or because he is excited, that he blushes because he is ashamed, that his tears flow because he is sad. This undeniable fact cannot be disputed, but it has to be explained by every theory denying a causal relation.

3. The third group comprises all the instances of one mental phenomenon being caused by another. There are three main cases to be considered. The first is what is generally known by the name of association. The second is the connection of intellect and will, or – on the level of sensible experience – of image and appetite. The third problem is of the relation of the lower and the higher faculties. In regard to this problem there are two main questions: the rôle played by sensible data in intellectual processes, and the relation of the sensitive appetite or – to use a modern term – of the "drives" and will.

The relations of ideas by association is doubtless, too, experienced as one of causality; we cannot describe these facts otherwise than by stating that something "made us think" of another thing. We form a conclusion because we had before thought of the premises. We are sure that one idea causes another to arise in our mind.

The problems of the psychology of association and of thought are of a particular interest here. The causal relations obtaining between two mental phenomena apparently represent the purest instance of mental causation. The study of perception and the one of action seem to be handicapped by the fact that in both instances one member of the causal relation belongs to another kind of reality. In thought or in association both are of the same kind. The central problem – which, indeed, will have to be discussed to some extent later – of the notion of quantity as applied to mental facts has to be studied first in regard to the causal relation of mental facts with each other.

The facts grouped under this head are furthermore important for the theory of causality in psychology because they make evident the necessity of introducing the notions of formal and of material cause. It is, indeed, impossible to give a satisfactory idea of the rôle played by the sensible image – the phantasma – in the evolution of abstract concepts unless one returns to the notion that the concept is caused by the activity of the *intellectus agens* and that the phantasma is accessory to this formation of a concept by acting as a material cause. The psychology of abstractive thought is, for that matter, one of the chapters of modern psychology where the ideas of the Schoolmen have been confirmed by experimental research; it is enough to recall the fine study Alex. Willwoll on "*Begriffsbildung*" published in 1926.

The relation of drive or instinct and will have been variously interpreted. It is, of course, not for this paper to give a detailed report on these theories. Most of them ignore the essential differences between an act of will and the experience of being pushed, as it were, by an instinctive craving. The psychoanalytical school of Freud is as guilty of such a neglect of manifest phenomenal data as is the theory of L. Klages. The first believes will to be but a modification of instinctive drives, the second conceives will as one instinct among others, *viz.*, as an instinct of inhibition. Many psychologists, without going so far as Freud, see will as a function which developed from instinct. This idea encounters the very same difficulties which form such a serious objection against all theories of evolution. It can not make any satisfactory statement on the process by which an undeveloped form ever may give rise to the appearance of a higher one, because it is unexplainable how some altogether new qualities may be created by evolution.

A psychology aware of the essential differences of will and instinct can not put up with such a theory. But it needs has to form an opinion on the relation of sensitive and intellectual appetite. Philosophy as well as a conscientious analysis of the facts converge towards the interpretation given by Aquinas (*e.g.*, I-II, q. 17, a. 4) : the act of a lower faculty is related to the act of the higher faculty as is matter to form. Will, indeed, gets hold, as it were, of the sensible appetite and uses it for its own ends.

Much could be said on the peculiarities of the problem of causality as it appears in the study of causal relations between mental states. But this would amount to a discussion of a quite undue length. We shall, moreover, take up this question once more.

4. The notion of mental faculty has been mentioned already. Psychology can not, indeed, do without it. One rather wonders at the criticisms brought forth against this notion. The very authors who are so much opposing it make use of it in other fields. The single "functions" physiology distinguishes are so many "faculties" of the body, "really distinct" from it and from each other.

No need, therefore, to justify the notion of faculty. By accepting it the psychologist is forced to face the question of the relation of the faculty and its single actual operations. The faculty is the "cause" of its acts, and it is necessary to give an account of (a) what is the peculiar nature of this causal relation, and (b) of the factors causing actualization.

This problem is partly but a special form of the more general one of the relation of *potentia* and *actus*, and is, therefore, not one of psychology alone. Its discussion is beyond the scope of this paper; but it had to be mentioned for sake of completeness and to show how manyfold, in fact, the problems referring to causality are.

The question of the relation of the faculties to each other has been touched upon already. There are, in this regard, of course, other questions besides those of the relation of the phantasma to the intellect or of the sensitive appetite to will. A thorough discussion would have to consider the place of intellect in regard to will, the one held by sensible data in regard to instinctive reactions, the relation of perception and imagination, and of both to memory, etc.

A peculiar difficult problem arises when one considers the relation of the vegetative faculties to the sensitive and the intellectual powers. The former represent the functional side of nearly all that is comprised today by the notions of constitution and heredity. These things are not only of a great actuality and very important in view of theory, they have also a definite bearing on many practical questions. No analysis of these problems can, however, be attempted without our previously having got a clear idea of the relation between body and mind.

5. Before turning to this central problem another has to be mentioned of which but a few words can be said. In accepting the notion of mental faculty psychology is forced to give an account of the relations obtaining between the faculties and the soul to which they belong. The statement that the faculties are "really distinct" from the soul and that they have to be considered as *accidentia propria* of the soul is too general as to supply a satisfactory answer. To give such an answer one would have to inquire into the general problem of the relations between accident and substance and to define more precisely the term of *accidentia propria. This is* again *a* thing not to be undertaken here; the problem had to be mentioned for sake of a complete survey.

6. Thus we arrive finally at the one question which is generally thought of whenever the notion of cause in psychology is mentioned:

the psychological problem, or the one of the relation of body and mind.

In the many discussions on this question a certain confusion reigns. The authors do not distinguish between the problem of the relation obtaining between mental and bodily phenomena and the other of the relation of body – or matter – to mind. This confusion is the effect of many of these authors adhering – even if they are not aware of doing it – to a kind of Platonic dualism. An interpretation, indeed, which considers body and mind as two separate substances which are but in touch with each other but do not form a real unity must give rise to the aforesaid confusion, because to such a theory the mental phenomena are exclusively effects of the soul's activity, the body being for nothing in them. But by failing to distinguish the two problems, the authors side, in a foregone conclusion, with a definite philosophy before they even have troubled to find out anything about the merits of this philosophy. Having once confused both problems, they are involuntarily led into some theory more or less like the one of the Platonists or into one which is a consequence of the former. The Platonic dualism, indeed, leads inevitably at considering mental phenomena as mere "epiphenomena"; there is, according to this view, no immediate influence either of the body on the mind, nor of the mind on the body. The machine-theory of the body as advocated by Cartesius is not less an offspring of Platonism than is the psychophysical-parallelism theory of G. Th. Fechner and his followers, or even the modern behaviorism; it is but logical to discard epiphenomena altogether, since they can have no influence on facts.

Even if it were not possible to show by way of an immanent critique that Platonic dualism is not in accordance with facts and not capable of explaining them satisfactorily, the latent self-contradictions of this theory alone would be sufficient to make it unacceptable. Nor seems it possible to invent a modification of this theory which could serve better.

There are but two views; one cannot think of another theory of the relations of body and mind but the one of Platonism and the other represented by Aristotelian-Thomistic hylemorphism. Materialistic monism is, of course, no theory of the psychophysical relation, because it denies the existence of one of the terms. Materialism is, by the way, another set of ideas which develops more easily from Platonism than from an Aristotelian philosophy, just because the former is always in danger of sublimating, as it were, the mental facts into mere epiphenomena.

By accepting the hylemorphic theory, psychology becomes capable of giving a satisfactory explanation of many facts. But there are still many difficulties. The general statement that the soul is the substantial form of the body, or, rather, of the human being, supplies only a platform from which to start, but it does not as yet allow to develop a theory of the special problems.

Nor is the hylemorphic conception altogether free from difficulties. Some arise from the principle of the *unitas formarum,* though those the opposite principle, of *pluralitas formarum,* brings about are doubtless more serious. One of the difficulties of the first kind is connected perhaps more with certain peculiarities of language than with such of conceptions. According to the strictly Thomistic theory we cannot well speak of relations of "body" and "soul," but only of those obtaining between matter and soul. "Body" is matter informed by the soul; there is no part and no function of the body which is not due to the informing and vivifying power of the soul. There are, moreover, but the purely intellectual acts of reason and will which are independent of matter, and we have, therefore, to bear in mind that many of our mental acts are in truth not acts of the immaterial soul alone but acts of the composite. We experience, however, our mental phenomena as being different in kind from those we call bodily. This is due, of course, to the peculiarities of the higher faculties and fits quite well with the hylemorphic conception; but it creates a definite difficulty of expression and even of thought.

The difficulties – a discussion of which would be too long – are, however, of no weight when compared to the enormous advantages of the hylemorphic conception. Only to point out a few of the latter: this theory eliminates all the difficulties in explaining the passing of an impulse from the body into the mind, since these both are conceived not as two separated substances which are but in touch with each other, but as a true composite, having but one nature. The bodily organ supplying to consciousness the sensible data is nothing outside of the mind, since it is matter informed by the soul. The same remark applies, of course, to the passing of an impulse from the mind into the body, *e.g.,* in the act of will. Another group of problems which becomes much clearer by applying to it the hylemorphic notion is the one falling under the head of terms as: constitution, heredity, types of body-built and character, *etc.*

The task of building up a self-consistent psychology on the basis of Aristotelian-Thomistic philosophy has still to be done; a thoroughly satisfactory psychology of this kind is still hard to find, if there is one at all.

After this indeed very fugitive survey of the problems concerning cause in psychology we may well ask whether cause is, when used in relation to mental phenomena, of the very same kind as we use it to describe relations of material facts. Even the very brief analysis of the problems concerning cause in psychology has shown that psychology needs all the "classical" forms of causality. Without introducing the notion of final cause no satisfactory theory of voluntary action can be devised; we cannot describe the process of abstraction unless we establish the materially causal relation of the phantasma in regard to the intellect; neither the true relation of instinct and will nor the one of matter and soul can be accounted for if the notion of formal cause is not accepted; the importance of efficient cause is too evident to need illustration.

It is, however, especially in regard to efficient cause that the question arises whether the notion of cause is univocally the same in every stratum of reality. It seems, indeed, that this is not the case.

There is a definite connection of efficient causality and quantity. If it can be shown that in psychology the notion of quantity has another sense than it has when applied to material facts, the presumption would gain in strength that the notion of causality, too, has a different meaning.

We will discard here the question of measurement in psychology; it would need a very thorough discussion, since there are evidently quite a few problems which are much in want of clarification. Even if the notion of measurement could be used in an univocal sense in psychology and in science, this would not as yet prove that quantity is a feature characteristic of every mental phenomenon as it is a basic feature of every material fact.

The causal relations between mental phenomena, especially those we comprise under the head of association and of discursive or syllogistic thought, are of a kind as to make the notion of quantity meaningless when applied to them. There are no grades of intensity in abstract notions or the thinking of them, nor can we think, e.g., the proposition of Pythagoras with a greater or a lesser intensity. There may be degrees of evidence – though the use of quantitative terms is probably but a metaphorical one – but it is impossible to find anything like differences of intensity in the thoughts themselves. The thought as such is always the same, and it has not more quantity than it has color.

But there is no doubt that causal relations exist also on the level of mere thought-processes. This, then, is an instance of causation without quantity being attached to the cause and to the effect. If, however, quantity loses its sense somewhat within the field of psychology, it becomes necessary to inquire into its use everywhere; maybe one would find out that the notion of quantity has within psychology but an analogous meaning and not univocally the same it is credited with on the level of matter.

The very moment the term of analogy is introduced psychology is forced to give up certain ideas which, indeed, are not its own at all, but which were taken over, without the necessary critique, from science. The psychologist is compelled, by the evidence of facts and the coercitive power of logical reasoning, to turn away from the modern – or still modern – conception of a thoroughgoing continuity; instead of assuming a series of transitions throughout the whole order of reality, he has to accept the idea of strata or levels existing together, related to each other, but nevertheless separated each from the other by an unbridgeable gulf. It is good to remember that the famous catchword *natura non facit saltus* is not the saying of a medieval philosopher but that it is contained in the works of the botanist Linnæus. Medieval philosophy conceived reality as a cosmos but not as a continuity.

We have simply to return to the old conception of a hierarchy of being and to apply the idea of *analogia entis* throughout this hierarchy.

As soon as one becomes aware of the merely analogical meaning of cause in psychology, many difficulties disappear and many problems are revealed as artificial and as due to a mistaken philosophy. The objections, for instance, which were raised in the name of the "unbroken chain of natural causes" against the assumption of free will become quite meaningless. The endeavors of certain physiologists – and so-called psychologists, too – to devise an "explanation" of mental facts in terms of biology lose all sense. Materialistic interpretation of mental life becomes impossible, because the very categories applicable to matter are not to be encountered in the level of mental phenomena.

What has been said here are, of course, but mere outlines and indications. Much work and much time will be needed to develop these preliminary remarks into a reliable theory of psychology.

We may, however, conclude that psychology supplies a strong argument in favor of retaining the "classical" notion of causality and its four forms. Physicists, whatever they may state on their own subject, are incapable of "dissolving" the notion of cause.

There is not only one problem of cause in psychology; there are several of them which have to be carefully distinguished for the sake of avoiding confusion. One has to beware especially from confusing the two problems of the relations obtaining between mental and bodily phenomena on one hand and of matter and soul on the other hand.

The hylemorphic conception proves to be the only one which supplies the basis for a self-consistent and satisfactory theory of psychology.

The categories of quantity and, accordingly, of causality have, on the level of mental facts, another meaning than they have on the one of material processes. A theory of psychology has to take account of the notions of a hierarchy of being and of the *analogia antis*.

Psychology thus depends in its theoretical foundation on metaphysics and ontology; on the other hand, it may supply to metaphysics some valuable data the latter may use for establishing still better its statements. Psychology thus serves metaphysics and is served by it. Psychology is not, perhaps, itself philosophy, but its relations to philosophy are at least closer than those of many of the other sciences.

To fulfill its very own tasks and to achieve its own perfection psychology needs has to become, what it essentially is: *ancilla philosophiæ*.

IRRESISTIBLE IMPULSES

A QUESTION OF MORAL PSYCHOLOGY

Many people refer to irresistible impulses as a valid excuse for some kind of misbehavior. Many a rash act is attributed to such impulses. Many an immoral deed is believed to be excusable because it allegedly sprang from strange and irresistible forces. The criminal will plead not guilty, on the claim that he did not really want to commit a crime, but became the victim of an irresistible impulse. And quite often the psychiatrist will confirm the statement of the defendant. As the criminal pleads not guilty in court, so do many people in the forum of their conscience and in the confessional. They do the same thing in private life when they have offended another or are criticized by others. The notion of irresistible impulses has found entrance into penal law; it has become generally recognized; everyone may avail himself of it. But this notion is far from being as clear and as well defined as one would wish it to be. Little is known about the criteria which may allow one to discover whether or not the statement of the culprit or the sinner is true. Unless we know more of these impulses, we may accept too easily the statement of these people that they "could not help it," or we may, on the other hand, be too ready to disbelieve them. It is therefore worth while to consider this problem.

The discussion shall be limited to normal persons, that is, to persons whose reason and will are not impaired by brain-trouble or by a real mental disease. The question of responsibility in insane people is much too complicated to be treated here.

There is, in a recently published book on *Honesty*, by Richard C. Cabot,[1] a remark which may well serve as a startingpoint of the discussion. Quoting from Wellman's works on the *Art of CrossExamination*, Dr. Cabot mentions a case in which the defendant had pleaded not guilty because of having acted under an irresistible impulse and the psychiatrist whom the judge asked to give his opinion confirmed the statement of the accused; thereupon the judge asked the psychiatrist, whether the accused would have acted in the same manner if a po-

1 Macmillan, New York, 1938, p. 269.

liceman had been present. The psychiatrist immediately replied in the negative. The judge concluded that the impulse seems to be irresistible in every case excepted in presence of a policeman. The judge, the scholarly author of the book on crossexamination, and Dr. Cabot himself evidently believe that an impulse to be irresistible has to be so under whatever circumstances. This idea, however, is far from being right.

Even reactions belonging to a lower level than true actions do depend on circumstances. Physiology used to define reflexes as automatic reactions following with absolute regularity the stimulation of some receptory field, and developing without the interference of consciousness and will. Though this definition holds good for the average case, it has nevertheless been shown to be too narrow and too much influenced by a merely mechanical conception of the living organism in general and the human being in particular. Physiology has discovered what some call today the "plasticity of the nervous reactions," Though the reflexes are due to the function of preëstablished anatomical structures and physiological functions, they may become modified by the general situation of the organism. Instinctive behavior in some animals is not only very complicated, but shows – notwithstanding the essential rigidity of instinctreactions – a certain plasticity and adaptability to circumstances. This is, of course, true in a still higher sense of human actions. It is quite possible for an impulse to be irresistible under certain circumstances and to become inhibited by other factors. The fact that the culprit would have not committed the criminal deed, had he been aware of the presence of a policeman, is no valid objection against his having acted under the pressure of an irresistible impulse. Irresistibility is not a fixed quality adhering to the impulse under all circumstances whatever and remaining unchanged when these circumstances are different. Not even a chemical process develops always in exactly the same manner, if the circumstances – as, e.g., temperature, acidity, concentration, etc. – become different. There is no reason to assume such an absolute constancy for impulses.

The man who committed a crime because unhappily no policeman was in sight, is not held back by the idea of law, of crime, of punishment, or of their visible representative, the policeman; for an idea or a memory is never as powerful as an immediate and actual impression. It is also quite probable that a man acting under such an impulse does not even for one short moment think of all these things. To have them in mind in a moment, where passion or some impulse becomes dominant, is only possible if a long training has been gone through previously and a habit has been developed. But one can hardly expect all people to develop conscientiously such a habit.

There are, perhaps, some impulses so powerful that they would overcome even the inhibitory force that the presence of a policeman may exercise. This may even be the case with a person whose mind is quite unimpaired; it is much more the case with one whose mind has been weakened by the action of some drug, be extreme fatigue, by long mental strain, or by momentary passion. Even in such a state a man may act apparently quite reasonably. The apparent reasonableness of behavior is indeed no objection against the assertion that the deed had been committed in an abnormal state of consciousness. We know that some patients may act reasonably, choose the appropriate means, execute some purposes, though their state of mind is definitely quite abnormal; this is observed, for instance, in cases of what is called crepuscular states in epileptics. Such a man may do quite complicated acts, travel for days, behave so that nobody even suspects his being mentally disturbed, and nevertheless he may be in an absolutely abnormal state of mind. There are also, within normality, certain states of monoideistic narrowing of consciousness, in which the subject may act quite reasonably in regard to his one dominant purpose, while no other thought can enter the mind and while, accordingly, no motives counteracting his idea ever can become efficient.

If we want to form an opinion on the irresistibility of a certain impulse, we have to consider not this impulse as such but the totality of the conditions, inner and outer, existing at the moment of action. The habit of isolating certain features of a situation – by which term we understand the totality of all subjective and objective features – and to treat them as if they were solid and immutable things, becomes definitely disastrous. A human action can be really understood only if it is viewed in its totality.

It is therefore impossible to declare, once and for all, that a given impulse is irresistible or that it is not. It may be irresistible, in the selfsane individual, one day and may not be so on another day. It is a truism to state, *si duo faciunt idem non est idem*. But is a too often neglected truth that the "same" action of one individual may have quite different motives, a different meaning, and carry a different responsibility each time it is executed. In the average we may, of course, rely on the constancy of motives and significations; but we should never forget that such changes may eventually take place. Every action, whether of two people or of the same person, has to be judged – by principle – separately and according to the conditions obtaining at the time it is done.

A person who is as a rule not subject to irresistible impulses may one day become the victim of one; an action we may, with good reason, believe to be due to the operation of such an impulse may, when repeated at another time, spring from free will or, at least, be not as irresistible as it was on a previous occasion. We may err on both sides, if we do not bear this fact in mind.

One has to distinguish the objective irresistibility of an impulse and the subjective conviction that such is the case. If this conviction is genuine, there is no great difference from the point of view of responsibility, but there is quite a marked one from the point of view of psychology, and there is one too in regard of "treatment," If a person is fully convinced of there being no chance of resistance, he will give way to an impulse even if it is not objectively irresistible. This is particularly true of impulses which, by their nature and their goals, are felt to be pathological or, at least, abnormal. It is a very common, though thoroughly mistaken, idea that a pathological impulse is irresistible *ipso facto*. This opinion is held not only by laymen, but also by many psychiatrists, physicians, moralists and confessors. It is justified neither by fact nor by philosophy. It is mostly due to a basically wrong conception of human nature. It is one of the great misfortunes of modern thought that there are so many heterogeneous and heretical ideas which nobody can avoid, and that these ideas, like a contagion, get hold also of minds which, by principle, are absolutely opposed to the philosophy responsible for these ideas. It is always useful to investigate the origin of ideas and to reveal their philosophical background.

The idea that it is enough for an impulse to be pathological to become irresistible is closely related to other conceptions which are generally, though not always consciously, accepted by the modern mind. Mankind today is manifestly unwilling to believe in the existence of sin. This unwillingness is not due to religious unbelief. Not sin as a theological notion is rejected, but the idea seems to have become unacceptable that man can, by his own free will, do the evil. This attitude goes back, probably, to Rousseau and the French Revolution. It is partly a reaction against the view of Protestant theology which declared human nature to be irreparably spoiled by original sin; not even Divine grace can repair the damage caused by the fall; it is God's mercy alone which, like a cloak, is laid over the essentially deformed soul, hiding its basic sinfulness. We see this kind of mentality still at work in Kant's idea that man is "radically" bad. The right balance, held so carefully by Catholic theology, the idea that man by original sin had become *spoliatus gratuitis, diminutus in naturalibus,* as it is put by the *Magister Sententiarum,* had been replaced by an extremely pessimistic notion. All extreme ideas have a tendency to bring forth, by way of reaction, their very opposite. Thus we see that, instead of the pessimistic conception of man's radical badness, in the mind of Rousseau – we should not forget that he grew up in Calvinistic Geneva – there arose the idea that man is "born good" and that all evil is due only to environmental factors. The notion of original sin, even as conceived by Catholic theology, is of course incompatible with this view. Much more incompatible is the Protestant idea. The century of Rousseau and the French Revolution saw the birth of a new "Humanism," a philosophy which made man the very centre and the summit of reality. Every wave of humanism that ever swept over the Christian world brought with it this incapacity to understand the notion of sin, especially original sin. This becomes very evident, for instance, to the student of the heresies of the twelfth century which in many of their aspects remind one of heresies of the sixteenth century.

If man is born good, his evil actions must spring from reasons alien to human nature. Sin, immoral behavior – or what to the modern mind becomes their equivalent: antisocial action – cannot be due to human nature itself. It has to be attributed to other factors, be they environmental forces or accidental modifications of human nature, like disease or the inheritance of pathological and abnormal characters. To safeguard the nobility and absolute supremacy of human nature these forces have to be subjected to irresistibility. If there existed still a small influence of intellect and will, the bad deed would again become the result of human nature itself. Human nature can be conceived as being essentially good only if either the idea of freedom is abandoned altogether or if it is, at least, rejected in the case of criminals, sinners or other wrongdoers. Materialistic mechanism and moral determinism could never have got hold of the modern mind, if the true notion of original sin – and, accordingly, of human nature – had not first been destroyed.

Thus, crime, misbehavior of every kind, moral defects have come to he considered as the effect of extrapersonal causes. Pathological impulses are, accordingly, viewed as being essentially irresistible, because otherwise the supremacy of human nature would suffer. The *mysterium iniquitatis* is indeed one of the strongest arguments in favor of a theocentric philosophy.

A man who believes his impulses to be irresistible because he feels them to be abnormal or because he has been told that they are, generally 'does not know of the reasons from which his belief springs. He may even adhere, and *bona fide* too, to a philosophy whose principles contradict his belief. We recall the case of a man, a Catholic, a teacher in a Catholic boarding school, who was addicted to some pederastic perversion and who sought help, because he trembled for his position and feared to get in conflict with the penal law. When he was asked why he did not refrain from his perverse acts, he was quite dumbfounded and replied: "How can I? These are abnormal impulses." He had never even thought of resisting, so strong was his conviction that all effort would be in vain, because abnormal impulses were, he believed, irresistible. When told that this was quite wrong he felt encouraged to attempt resistance; he was amazed to discover that he need not yield to the impulses.

Why, indeed, should anyone suppose that, a homosexual impulse, for instances, is essentially irresistible, when we expect people to resist the normal impulses of sexuality? Unless a homosexual is – which indeed is the case with several of them – a thoroughly abnormal personality whose perversion is but one symptom of a general neurosis, he is as capable of refraining from indulging in his abnormal sexual impulses as a normal person is in face of heterosexual impulses.

The abnormality of an impulse as such is not a proof of irresistibility and therefore not a valid excuse. It presents, moreover, the danger of confusing what may be but a strong temptation or attraction with a real impulse.

Irresistibility may result from two factors that should be carefully distinguished, because the psychological background is different in each of them. The overpowering strength of the impulsive situation may arise from the force of the impulse or from the knowledge that by not giving way to it some other phenomena are sure to occur which are felt to be intolerable. In the second case the irresistibility is not from the impulse itself but accidental to it, though not less effective. This is observed, for example, in many cases of compulsory neurosis: the patient knows that he is capable of offering resistance to the impulse, at least for a time, but that by doing so he will bring about, say, an unsupportable fit of anxiety, or he fears that the idea of not doing the thing will stay on and incapacitate him for doing anything. He foresees that he will have to give in anyhow, and thus it is much simpler to do it the moment the impulse is felt.

Many of these impulses, especially in compulsory neurosis, seem to be, at first sight, morally indifferent. There is nothing bad in picking up every scrap of paper, or of returning seven tines to make sure that the door is really locked, or in touching three times every object before letting it go. But even these apparently harmless things have a bearing on morality. They cause an enormous loss of time; they often become a serious handicap in fulfilling one's duties; and, last not least, they upset the scale of values of things, since merely subjective things are credited with a quite undue importance. No human action is quite indifferent from the moral point of view, and this fact becomes very plain in such cases as these.

Another necessary distinction is the one between irresistibility caused by the mere strength of the impulse and the one arising from the alleged intolerability of the situation which is going to be changed by obeying the impulse. The first case is seen in certain actions caused by passion: in a fit of violent anger it is the strength of the aggressive impulse which overpowers all the other faculties. The second case is evident in many sexual acts: the impulse is not the most important feature in the whole situation; it is the great tension, the craving for relief which is not to be resisted.

These irresistible impulses are observed, probably only in cases of violent passion. In nearly all the other cases we have to deal with overstrong attraction or with experiences which are felt to be intolerable. In these latter cases the phenomenon of irresistibility is much more complicated than appears at first sight. Most of the stories about cases of irresistibility tell of the fact that the person "could not resist any longer," that he "finally had to give in," These words show that the impulse was not of a kind to rush the individual headlong, as it were, toward a certain goal. They imply furthermore that something like consent and decision took place. Resistance had to be abandoned before the impulse could become really irresistible. Yielding is after all an act of will, and so is, for that matter, not resisting at all. Only in those cases in which the impulse arises so suddenly and with such strength as not to allow for consciousness, for some deliberation, however brief, or for the attempt to, at least, delay action, there is really no act of will at all. It seems that these cases are limited to acts caused by an overwhelming passion, anger, fury, despair, or fear. In all other cases there is, as it seems, left at least some little bit of freedom.

This fact makes the decision on responsibility very difficult, all the more since there are no reliable objective criteria of irresistibility. We know only what the individual himself sees fit to tell us. Even if we feel sure of his sincerity, we never can know whether he remembers correctly the whole fact. His memory may be unreliable. This is not improbable, for details of troubling experiences are apt to become forgotten, and because the mind, involuntarily, fills in the gaps of memory. There is moreover the tendency of finding plausible excuses for actions at which we feel ashamed, and this tendency may be at work even without our noticing it.

There is no impulse which may be considered simply as irresistible. We know no qualities whose presence would make it sure that a given impulse had been irresistible or, for that matter, [216] that it had been not of such a kind. It is sometimes asserted that actions which need a longer preparation or a series of preliminary steps cannot be due to the influence of an irresistible impulse; we have already mentioned facts which disprove this idea. The fact of sudden and violent action may become a strong argument in favor of irresistibility having existed; but the absence of this feature is no convincing proof to the contrary.

It all depends therefore on the reliability of the subject himself. A judgment on such facts is possible only if we sufficiently understand the total personality. The confessor may start with the presumption of credibility and sincerity, as a man going to confession will probably want to be sincere. It is surely permissible to apply the principle *in dubiis mitius*. The problem becomes much more difficult when the confessor has to attempt to reform his penitent and if the latter seriously desires to get rid of actions for which he feels not responsible, but which he knows nevertheless are wrong.

The first thing to do is probably to warn the penitent that irresistibility, even it can be proved in some cases, is not to be assumed for all of them, regardless of the circumstances. We cannot let the penitent believe that he has got an excuse which will hold good once and for all.

There are several ways of dealing with these irresistible impulses. One may advise a person who complains of such troubles to avoid as far as possible the situations which favor their arising. As a rule this isn't easy and it cannot be done at all in many cases. Sometimes a man may foresee that he will become the victim of an impulse if he lets things develop; he may know, for instance, that a dispute will make him angry and that, within a short time, he will not be able to control his temper; he may learn to quit the argument, even at the cost of appearing beaten or a coward. Unhappily, most people do not know when to run away; it is the same thing with sexual temptations too.

There is one very curious and very important feature worthy of mention in those irresistible impulses. They become irresistible, so to say, before they have fully developed. People have a presentiment of the impulse arising; they know that within a short time they will become entangled in a situation from which there is no escape, much as they may desire one. They know that they are still capable, this very moment, of turning away and that by doing so they will avoid the danger – but they do not. There is a peculiar fascination, a lurid attraction in this kind of danger, and there is evidently some anticipation of the satisfaction that the *partes inferiors animae* will derive from indulging in the "irresistible" action. This action itself may, therefore, not carry any responsibility and nevertheless not be excusable, because in fact the person has assented to its development.

But a man may become, little by little, master of these impulses if he cares to think of them and to prepare for them in times when they are not present. Here too, as in many other cases, the word of St. Ignatius Loyola applies, that it is the *tempus quietum* during which we make progresses.

An irresistible impulse is not always the effect of some pecularity of constitution or temperament; it may be conditioned by some mental attitudes which are unknown to or not understood by the person himself. Some modern schools of psychology speak of the working of the "unconscious." It is well to avoid this term, because of its vagueness, unless its meaning is exactly defined. To do this would, however, necessitate a wide analysis. The socalled unconscious motives, tendencies, forces, etc. are really – at least with many people – not so unconscious after all; it needs often only a little explanation to make them see what is the matter with them. Many of the irresistible impulses rest not on factors of constitution but on acquired habits – understanding the term in the sense of scholastic psychology – of which the individual is not aware and whose true nature he does not realize. The discovery of hidden motives or habits is, however, the task of the psychologist or even the psychiatrist rather than the spiritual director.

The confessor needs, as it seems, to be careful not to encourage the penitent to continue with his habit by telling him that he is acting under the influence of an irresistible impulse. The penitent interprets this statement easily as a kind of permission to act as he is doing and not to care, because he is not responsible and does not commit a *peccatum formale*. Tiresome though it may be, one will have to inquire over and over again into the peculiar circumstances and to find out each time anew whether there has been an irresistible impulse or not. Only if one knows the personality of the penitent very well and has good reasons for trusting him, and after it has been ascertained that the immoral actions were indeed due always to such an impulse, one may dispense the penitent from reporting every instance.

Many cases of this kind have to be classed simply among those of compulsory neurosis. These cases have to be treated. Ordinarily, it is not for the priest to deal with them. He will have to tell them that they are just abnormal personalities, that there are ways to help them and that they are, if it can be done, morally obliged to seek the advice of a trustworthy psychiatrist.

There is a danger in believing that one is the victim of an irresistible impulse. Even if the actions due to it are not sinful, because done without the person really willing them, there is always the danger of these persons enlarging – unwillingly, apparently, but nevertheless not without a certain responsibility – the field of action of these impulses. They will describe the fact by saying that things have become worse with them, implying that their abnormal state has gained in intensity or in extension. It is, however, improbable that an impulse which for a long time has been limited to a definite kind of behavior, should spread into fields often very different. In such cases there is need of great caution.

It is, on the other hand, necessary to encourage many of these people. Quite a few suffer intensely from the idea that they are committing sins over and over again. Although they may feel that they are not fully responsible, they nevertheless feel too that these actions are not forced on them by powers altogether outside their own personality. They may despair of their eternal fate, of their ever being able to lead a moral life, and thus be induced to give up trying to live religiously. Even if they do not go so far, they may give up all striving for perfection and thus gradually sink to lower and lower levels of morality. They have to be told, however, not only that, so long as these impulses are really irresistible, there is no grave sin; they have to be told also that even irresistible impulses may be dealt with somehow. It is necessary to find a middle way between letting these people believe that they have a privilege to ignore certain commandments and discouraging them by open disbelief or harshness.

The most important thing is that every ease is to be considered as an altogether new problem, and that one must strictly avoid all generalization, most of all of a rashly formed opinion. We cannot know anything of the true nature of the allegedly irresistible impulse unless we know all we can find out about the total personality. Neither the psychiatrist nor the confessor has to deal with the isolated phenomenon of an impulse: both deal with a human person whom the impulse seizes.

THE VIS COGITATIVA AND EVALUATION

Many misunderstandings between the modern, experimental, and the Scholastic, introspective psychologies arise from the fact that both speak different languages and that the one does not know the meaning of the term used by the other. It is enough, to illustrate this state of things, to remember the significations of the terms "imagination" and "memory" in St. Thomas and in experimental psychology. If both parties would trouble to make sure of the meaning they have in their minds, they doubtless might come to some agreement. Sometimes, the disagreement is not with the terms but with the interpretation of certain facts. The theory of perception or the ideas on Gestalt not only allow for, but make even necessary the *sensus commis;* pathology too points in the same direction.[1] I have tried to show that the controversy on "imageless thought" is mostly due to such a mutual misunderstanding, the experimentalists not knowing what the Scholastic psychologists refer to when they speak of the indispensability of the phantasm in forming and using the abstract notion, and the Scholastics being ignorant of the facts discovered by experimental psychology.[2]

Among the sensory faculties listed by Thomistic psychology there is one which to the experimental psychologist probably, appears as a mere construction: the *vis æstimativa v. cogitativa.* Empirical psychology does not know what to do with this faculty which apparently it does not need and, therefore, considers as an unnecessary and unfounded construct. That is, the psychologists would hold this opinion, if they knew of this faculty at all. But they do not know of it, because to them certain problems which may necessitate the introduction of this faculty do not arise within the framework of categories supporting today's psychologies.

1 Cf. Th. V. Moore, *Cognitive Psychology,* Chicago, 1939.

2 R. Allers, "The Intellectual Cognition of Particulars," *The Thomist,* 1941, 111, 95.

A closer study of certain empirical data collected by the experimentalists on one hand and an analysis of the true meaning of the Scholastic conception, however, may serve to prove that (a) the notion of the *vis cogitativa* is well founded, (b) not at all contrary to the findings of psychology, and (c) even of such a kind that it can be profitably used in empirical psychology.

This article is concerned with studying only one aspect of the problem, namely the relation of the *vis cogtativa* to the facts known in regard to the awareness of values. This question seems to be particularly suitable for demonstrating the use psychology may make of the Scholastic notion and also for clarifying one of the many points still problematic in. the theory of this internal sense.

The relations of the *vis cogitativa* to the other internal senses and the questions whether, how far, and in what way the *vis cogitativa* co-operates in forming the phantasm on which the active intellect may work, are discarded. Nor will the problem be considered whether the "general image" is an. achievement of imagination alone or whether it is, as its quasi-conceptual nature suggests, due to the influence of the *vis cogitativa*.

Because of this limitation of the problem it seems permissible to ignore the important and interesting explanations given by Cajetanus and Ferrariensis. The discussions of these authors concern mostly the relation of the sensory faculties and the intellect; they focus on the problems of the formation and the development of the phantasm and its rôle in the disengaging of the -universal nature from the particular image.

I

In animals, there is, we read in St. Thomas, a capacity of apprehending certain data which are not immediately and as such given by the external senses. The classic example to which Aquinas repeatedly refers is the one of the sheep being aware of the dangerousness of the wolf. What they sense is merely a shape, a size, a color, the sound of the howl. Dangerousness is nothing which appears immediately in these features. Nor is the awareness of favorable or unfavorable environmental factors acquired by experience; we see even the young animal behaving in a suitable manner. There is no rational capacity in animals; they can not conclude in any way from the sense-data that what they apprehend is indicative of danger. One has, therefore, to assume that the brutes are gifted with a particular faculty enabling them to become cognizant of favorable and unfavorable environmental situations. This faculty is given the name of *vis æstimativa*.

Modern authors often translate this term by "instinct." But instinct as used by psychologists to-day means more than a cognitive faculty. By instinct biology and psychology refers to a complex function determining a certain type of behavior. Instinct is not only what sets such a mechanism going, but also the power behind the "instinctive" action. The *vis aestimativa* accordingly, corresponds only to the cognitive or, to speak the language of physiology, the afferent part of the total instinctual mechanism. In the terminology of St. Thomas *instinctus* means indeed what releases the activity of the sensory appetites. But it is somewhat confusing to see in modern texts this term used in a sense not any longer generally accepted.

The *vis æstimativa* is considered by St. Thomas as the highest faculty existing in the animal organism; it comes close to reason (*attingit rationem*).[3] In man its achievements become still greater and more like those of reason, wherefore this power is called *vis cogitativa* or *ratio particularis*. The "closeness" to the rational faculties and, generally speaking, it being rooted in a rational soul "enobles" this power and raises it above the level it attains in brutes. This, however, must be true of the other sensory faculties too, though the difference between the human and the animal faculties may not be as apparent as it is in the case of the *vis cogitativa*. The "nobilitation" of the sensory-and even, perhaps of the vegetative-is based, first, on the rationality of the soul to which all these faculties belong, and secondly on a direct and directing *refluentia* or influence of the intellect and will on the performances of the senses. Rational will makes use of the appetites for realizing its proper end, the universal good, in the particular instances. Intellect plays a determining rôle in sense-perception, since the mere recognizing of a thing perceived as one of this or that kind implies the consciousness of an universal. The well known facts which illustrate the influence of knowledge and intellectual interpretation on sense-perception, certain experimental data, which however can not be reported here, and other instances prove too that the influence of the rational faculties penetrates far into processes which, at first sight,

---

3 *In III Sent.*, d. 26, q. 1, a. 2c.

appear to be purely physiological."[4] It is, therefore, true that one may distinguish two forms of activity of the *vis cogitativa,* one after, and one before the intellect has been actuated.[5]

Our knowledge of the mental operations in animals is only an indirect one. We conclude from animal behavior the existence and the mode of functioning of certain faculties we discover within ourselves. Even the notion of "behavior" is originally developed from self-experience. The direct knowledge -we have of our own mind and its performances remains, inevitably, the starting point and the basis even of the most "objective" psychology, even of behavorism. As soon as psychology wants to be more than a mere description of reactions to definite environmental situations, it has to refer to self-experience. If we wish to make some statement on the mental functions underlying "behavior," it is introspection which furnishes the clues. If this is to be called anthropomorphism, than psychology is condemned for ever to be anthropomorphous. Under these circumstances, it is preferable to limit psychological discussions to the evidences we get from the study of the human mind, and to leave animal psychology besides. The following pages deal, accordingly, only with the *vis cogitativa* as a faculty of the rational soul.

To understand the nature of the *vis cogitativa,* one has to make clear, first, what are its proper objects, secondly, what are its relations to the other, sensory and rational, faculties.

The object of this power is the **particular** end or good;[6] certain *commoditates et utilitates sive nocumenta;*[7] the *intentiones quae per sensum non accipiuntur.*[8] Statements like the last led later authors to speak of the objects of the vis *cogitativct* as *in,sensala* or '*intentiones insensatae.*[9]

---

4 Some pertinent observations may be found in R. Allers, "Uebur einige Untersechiede des ein- und des beidaeugigen Sehens," *Sitz. Ber. Wiener Akad. Z. d. Wiss. Naturwiss. Klasse,* 1935, CXLIV, p. 33 and R. Allers u. E. Schoemer, Ueber den "Wettstreit der Hoerfelder," *ibid.,* p. 401.

5 G. P. Klubertanz, "The Internal Senses in the Process of Cognition," *The Modern Schoolman,* 1941, XVIII, 29.

6 *Summa Theol.,* I-II, q. 11, a. 2e.

7 *Summa Theol.,* I, q. 78, a. 4e.

8 *Ibid.*

9 E. g., Joannes a St. Thoma, *Cursus Phiosophicus,* ed. Reiser, Taurin., 1937, Vol. III, p. 385, b. 14 (IV, q. 12, a, 1).

The "commodities," etc., apprehended by the *vis cogitativa* are, however, not objects of the same kind as the data of the external senses. It is a commodity for us (or for any organism which apprehends it), therefore a relation. Because of this internal sense is said to be *collativa intentiortnum particularium*[10] 15 and, since combining and dividing is a capacity characteristic mostly of the intellect, also *ratio particularis.*[11] The right estimation of a particular end may be even called *intellsctus* "insofar as it is of some principle, and sense insofar as it is particular. And this what the Philosopher says in VI. Eth. e. 11: singulars, are necessarily apprehended by the sense; this however is in the intellect. One has, however, to understand this not as asserted of the particular sense by which we know the properly sensibles, but of the internal sense by means of which we judge on particulars."[12] Thus, it seems as if the only proper objects of the *vis cogitativa* were certain particular goods, or certain values actually existing in some things, related to notions like convenience, usefulness, dangerousness, and suchlike. It is, however, hardly possible to restrict the operation of this sensory power to the values only of the types mentioned before. The rational will can not consider any particular object without some intermediary function which forms, a it were, the connecting link between the immaterial faculty and the material particular in which the values, as realized and desirable or as to be realized by man's action, 'reside. Now, there are many values which do not belong to the classes of usefulness, convenience, damage, or danger. These values too must be brought close to the will by some intermediary, which naturally can not be any other than the *vis cogitativa*. We shall have, therefore, to conclude that other kinds of value too are apprehended by this interior sense. It

10 *In IV Eth.*, 1. 1 Ca. fin.

11 *In I Met.*, **1. 1.**

12 II-II, q. 49, a. 2 ad 3um. Most of the terminology in this matter seems to be taken from the Latin translations of the Arabian philosophers. The expressions *vis aestimativa, cogitativa, ratio,* and *collatio* occur in Avicenna, Alfarabi, and Averroës and are need also by St. Albert who refers to this power as capable of election, of apprehending the convenient and the inconvenient. *Cogitativa quae est actus rationis conferentis de perticularibus.* A. Schneider, *Die Psychologie Albert des Grossen,* Muenster, 1903, p. 165 (Beitr. z. Gesch. d. Phil. d. MA. 5, H. 3-5). The use of *cogitativa* for the human faculty and *æstimativa* for the power in brutes is equally found in Avicenna and Alfarabi.

is the more necessary to credit the *vis cogitativa* with such a capacity, since the universal notion of values – e.g., of moral values – can not be imagined developing, unless there be some sense supplying the substratum from which the general notion may be disengaged.

St. Thomas, when explaining the functions of the *vis cogitativa* usually refers to illustration taken from animal life. Also, he speaks only of the *convenienia v. nocumemtun* becoming known by actual sense-impressions, originating from an object present. It is, however, clear that phantasms or images must also be capable of serving as a source to this internal sense. In deciding upon some future action, deliberating on its goodness, and contemplating several possible aims, we deal not with objects actually present. We contemplate several possibilities of how the actual situation may be changed by our future actions. The various situations, eventually to be brought about by our doing, are envisioned in imagination, founded upon the actually apprehended situation and previous experience. The images are not "copies," but "constructs." But in them we distinguish degrees and differences of goodness, which performance belongs, since these values are incorporated in images referring to particular situations, to the *vis cogitativa.*

It seems, therefore, correct to define the proper object, in this regard, of the *vis cogitativa* as any value whatsoever, in so far as it is realized in a particular thing or a particular situation and apprehended as such.

In any organism things are arranged that way that the lower functions serve the higher, and that the higher serve the whole. The senses serve reason, and will makes use of the sensory appetites as well as of the vegetative and locomotive faculties, so that man may attain its true ends. Such a view sounded quite strange to the minds of biologists and psychologists but a short time ago. But nowadays many of them are reverting to conceptions which, although hardly stated in the same terms, are in truth but little different from the notion of the organism as a hierarchy of functions governed by some intrinsic principle. The name given to this principle is another with every school and nearly every scholar. They call it Entelechy, or a principle of *Gestalt,* or they speak somewhat darkly of the wholeness of an organic structure or of an organism; but they refer to what has been known since ages as the *forma substantialis.*

It does not matter what terms are used. The main thing is that even biology and psychology can not help acknowledging that there is some unifying principle in the organism, that there are higher and lower functions, higher and lower performances, and, that any impairment of the former lowers the total achievements of the organism to a level similar to the one held by less perfect organisms.

The idea that the higher functions in an organism, or the higher organisms in the totality of living beings, are "nothing but" complex manifestations of the most simple and most elementary functions and beings we observe, has to be given up, and has been given up already by some of the leading authorities. It is, therefore, not necessary any longer to defend and to justify at length a conception which holds that the lower functions exist for the sake of the higher. The senses are there for the rational faculties, and not the latter for the sake of the former. This applies to the internal senses and the sensory appetites as it does to the external senses and the vegetative or locomotive faculties.

The hierarchy of faculties, however, has not to be conceived as if the single faculties possessed any real independence or operated irrespectively of the whole to which they belong. St. Thomas is careful to enjoin that it is not the faculty which operates, but the human person operates by means of the faculties. Since the ultimate aims of man are conceived in his intellect which presents them to rational will, it is evident that there has to be a twofold relation of the sensory and the rational faculty. The senses supply the intellect with the material from which to develop the universal notions; but there is also a directing influence of the intellect on the sensory performances:

How this directing influence of the intellect comes to reach the sensory faculties it not easy to say. The statements of St. Thomas in this regard are brief and without further explanations. There is, we are told, a twofold mode of action in any agent; "one according to the agent's own nature, and another according to the nature of the higher agent. The impression, namely, of the higher agent remains in the lower and, because of this, the lower agent acts not only by way of its own action, but also of the action of the higher agent."[13]

After having commented on the '*reflexio* super phantasma which enables the immaterial intellect to get hold, indirectly, of the material particular, St. Thomas proceeds: "There is another mode (sc. than the knowing of the particular) according to which the movement which

13 *Q. d. de Ver.*, q. 22, a. 13c: ... *uno modo secundum quod competit suae naturae, alia modo secunclum quod competit naturae superioris agentis. Impressio enim superioris agentis manet in inferiori, et ea hoc inferius agens non solum agit notione propria sed actione superioris agentis.*

starts from the soul towards the things begins in the mind (*mens*, here evidently, as one sees from the preceding, synonymous with intellect) and proceeds into the sensitive part, insofar as the mind rules over the inferior powers and such gets mixed up with the singulars by the mediation by the particular reason which is a certain individual power, also called by the name of *cogitativa*."[14]

Much the same idea is expressed, also in *de Veritate*, differently. The receptive as well as the orective powers of the sensitive part determine the operations of the sensible soul; but, on the other hand, the sensitive soul" has some modest participation of reason, the lowest part of which it (the sensitive soul) touches with its highest."[15] One has to admit that this statement is not without difficulties. It is hard to see how the "highest part" of the sensory faculties, which are essentially material, and have, as St. Thomas repeatedly remarks, definite organs in which they reside, can "get in touch" with the immaterial faculty. The term of *continuatio* which St. Thomas occasionally rises in this connection does not contribute much to the clarification of the problem. This problem, however, is concerned not only with the relation of the *vis cogitativa* and the intellect, but generally with the relations between sensory and rational faculties. It has to be discussed on a broader basis. But it may be mentioned that, according to Aquinas, the link which connects the rational and the sensory faculties is just the *vis cogitativa*. Thus, an elucidation of the nature of this power may serve, in some way, as a preliminary study, preparing the terrain for a more thorough investigation.

As to the intellect, so is the *ratio particularis* related also to the rational will. It has been remarked before that there has to be some intermediary between the particular object, in which the general intention of will is to be realized, and the will itself, the one being immaterial and the other material. The decision on a particular action is described by St. Thomas as a syllogism in. which the maior is a general proposi-

14 *Q. d. de Ver.*, q. 10, a. 5c: ... *alio modo secundum quod motus qui; est ab anima ad res incipit a mente et procedit in partem sensitivam, prout mens regit inferiores vires, et sic singularibus se immiscet mediante ratione particulari quae est potentia quaedam individualis quae alio nomine dicitur cogitativa.*

15 *Q d. de Ver., q. 25, a. 2c: ... tam ex parte apprehensivarum virium quam cx parte appetitivarum sensitivae partis aliquid competit sensibili animae secundum propriam naturam; aliquid vero secundum habet aliquam modicam participationem rationis, attingens ad ultimum eius in sui supremo.*

tion and the minor one about a particular. The latter is supplied by the *ratio particularis*. In animals, it is the æstimative power which moves the appetites. "In. the place of the æstimative power man possesses, as has been said before (I. q. 78. a. 4. c.) the *vis cogitativa* which some call *ratio particularis*, because it is capable of bringing together the individual intentions. It is thus the nature of the human sensitive appetite to be moved by this power. It is the property of the *ratio particularis* itself to be moved and directed according to the meaning of universals; therefore, conclusions regarding singulars are drawn in syllogisms from universal propositions."[16] Because the conclusions regarding singulars are achieved not by the intellect, but by this ratio, the sensory appetite obeys more the latter than the intellect proper.[17]

In this statement is implied a notion which offers even a greater difficulty than the one mentioned before. It is sufficiently difficult to see how a sensory faculty can actually get in touch with an immaterial one, or how the latter may leave its imprint in the former. But here, we have to do with the result of a purely intellectual operation, namely the universal proposition, being taken over by the *vis cogitativa*. The conclusions about singulars are performed by the *ratio particularis* therefore both the maior and the minor have to be present in this faculty. But, if it is impossible for the intellect to get hold directly of a particular, it is still more impossible for the material faculty to include in one operation both the universal proposition worked out by the intellect, and the particular which proceeds from the activity of the particular reason itself.

Not only the particular reason, also the *appetitus* itself is said to participate somehow in the nature of the higher, rational faculty. There is a perfect symmetry in this. To the intellect corresponds, on the sensory level, the *vis cogitativa*; to the rational will, the appetite, insofar as

16 *Summa Theol.*, I, q. 81, a. 3c. *Loco autem aestimativae virtutis est in homine, sicut supra dicitur, vis cogitativa quae dicitur a quibusdam ratio particularis eo quod est collativa intentionum individualium. Unde ab ea natus est moveri appetitus sensitivus. Ipsa autem ratio particularis nata est moveri et dirigi secundum rationem universalium unde in syllogisticis ex universalibus propositionibus concluduntur conolusiones singulares.*

17 *Ibid ... deducere universalia principia in conolusiones singulares non est opus simplicis intellectus sed rationis; ideo irascibilis et concupiscibilis magis dicuntur obedire rationi quam intellectui.*

it is directed towards an apprehended and known particular good.[18] There is even such an expression as *voluntas sensualitatis.*[19]

There is another interpretation which does not simplify the problem either, but only locates it, instead in the sensory, in the rational faculty. "The intellect or the reason knows in the universal the end towards which it ordains the act of the concupiscible and the irascible appetites, by commanding them. This universal knowledge it applies to the singular by means of the *vis cogitativa.*[20] This reads as if the particular proposition, achieved by or in the *vis cogitativa* were in some way transmitted to the intellect, and as if it were the intellect which draws the conclusion regarding the singular. It seems as if St. Thomas himself had not felt quite sure which solution to adopt. One is not wrong, probably, in assuming that Aquinas had not reached a definite and satisfactory answer to the question of the relation and the co-operation between the sensory and the intellectual faculties. It seems also as if the *attingere ralionem, of which he speaks in regard to the vis cogitative.* were a somewhat ambiguous term. In the passages quoted above the statements on the closeness of the internal sense to the intellect is made in regard to the human mind; there these two faculties in fact work side by side and influence each other mutually. But St. Thomas uses the same expression also in regard to the *vis æstimativa* in animals. And here the factor of closeness or of belonging to the same soul can not enter into play. The expression that "the sensitive part apprehends those intentions which do not fall under the sense according to its attaining reason"[21] can refer only to a close similarity of nature. This meaning, however, gives no sense when reference is made to the human mind, because mere similarity is no explanation of the cooperation of the two faculties.

There are two ways of co-operation possible. The one is represented by the imaginations supplying the intellect with the phantasm. The

18 *In III Sent.*, d. 17, q. 1, a. 1, sol. 2; d. 26, q. 1, a. 2c

19 *In II Sent.*, d. 17, q. 1, a. 2, q. 3c.

20 *Q. d. de Ver.*, q. 10, a. 5 ad 4um. *Intellectus s. ratio cognoscit in universali finem ad quem ordinet actum ooncupiscibilis et actum irascibilis imperando eos. Hanc autem cognitionem universalium mediante vi cogitativa ad singularia applicat.*

21 *In III Sent.*, d. 26, q. 1, a. 2c ... *quod apprehendit (animal) illas intentiones quae non cadunt suo sensu ... hoc est sensitivae panis secundum quod attingit rationem.*

other consists in an active co-operation, both co-operating faculties tending towards the same end. Of this kind of co-operation of intellect and particular reason seems to be, since both have to be active for the mind to arrive at a particular conclusion. This contradicts somewhat the statement that of two powers of the soul, when operating at the same time, the one necessarily hinders or even inhibits the other.[22] That this statement is according to fact is beyond any doubt; it is also confirmed by many experimental results. Only, it hardly can be asserted in complete generality that there is only mutual inhibition and not also mutual furthering. The notions, reported before, on the cooperation of the intellect and the *vis cogitativa*. on one hand, the *vis cogitativa* and the will on the other imply such a mutual furthering. Also of this we have experimental evidence; there are furthermore certain common experiences one may mention. Everybody knows, e.g., that certain, people think better when walking around, which means that the activity of the locomotor faculty has a favorable influence on the performances of the intellect. Or one may refer to the fact that emotions, under certain conditions, help a man in finding some solutions, whereas under other conditions they exercise a definitely inhibiting influence. Sometimes, a man will find a way out of a difficult situation under the pressure of necessity, while he would not hit on the idea when emotionally undisturbed. And so on.

It seems necessary to distinguish between operations going on in two faculties both aiming at the same goal, and others which, because of different intention, hinder the one the other. In regard to the first case, there is the help lent by imagination to the intellect not only in abstraction, but also when clarifying some abstract notion by means of illustrations. Or the appetites putting, as it were, to the disposal of rational will their particular energy.

It is not within the scope of the present article to attempt a solution of the difficulties pointed out above. They had to be mentioned not to let the opinion arise that the system of St. Thomas is fully perfected in every detail, and the task of the psychologist trained in Scholastic philosophy consists simply in either fitting the findings of experimental research into the ready-made framework of Thomistic psychology, or to reject these findings as contradicting this system.

One of the main functions of the *vis cogitativa*, according to St. Thomas, has doubtless to do with the cognition of values as realized

22 *Summa Theol.*, I-II, q. 77, a. lc.

actually or possibly, in particular things and situations, and with the adjustment, so to say, of the will to particular ends. As ends of human action and as objects of human appreciation values are founded on the relation with the individual person apprehending these values or purposing this or that action. This, however, does not imply that values consist in or am founded upon exclusively in such a relation to a human person and have no being outside of such a relation. Some more will be said on this later.

If one is right in supposing that St. Thomas himself did not consider his system as complete and closed, one may justly ask whether the description he gives of the functions of the *vis cogitativa* is exhaustive or whether there are not other performances which may be attributed to this power. When speaking of the *vis cogitativa,* St. Thomas nearly regularly refers to values as the objects. Sometimes, however, he seems to imply that the functions of this power are not limited to only these objects. E. g. he declares that the "act of the *vis cogitativa* consists in combination and division,"[23] without giving any specification, just in one of the fundamental passages. The same sweeping statement is to be found in the Commentary on Eth. VI.[24] and in the one on Met. 1.[25] Less clear is another passage: "The disposition of the wise in regard to singulars is achieved by the mind (intellect) only by the intermediary of the *vis cogitativa* to which devolves the cognition of the singular intentions." [26] It is probable that the term *intentio* means simply object; but it might also refer to ends of the orective powers.

These passages encourage a wider interpretation of the functions attributed to the *vis cogitativa*. This is also the opinion of C. Fabro[27] and

23 *Summa Theol.,* I, q. 78, a. 4. *Actus cogitativae qui est conferre et componere et dividere.*

24 *In VI Eth.,* 1. 1. *Alio modo possunnt accipi contingentia, seccundum quod sunt in particutari et sic variaiUa sunt nec cadit super sa inteilectus nisi mediante potentiis sensitivis. Unde inter partes animae sensitivae ponitur una potentia quae dioitur ratio particularis.*

25 *In I Met.,* 1. 1. *Experimentum enim est ex collatione plurium singularium in memoria receptorum. Huiusmodi collatio est homini propria et pertinet ad vim cogitativam.*

26 *Q, d. de Ver.,* q. 10, a. 5 ad 2um.

27 C. Fabro, "Knowledge and Perception in Aristotelic-Thomistic Psychology," *The New Scholasticism,* 1938, XII, 337.

of G. P. Klubertanz.[28] The latter speaks of the discursive operation in the *vis cogitativa* and evidently has in mind more than the mere awareness of usefulness or danger and the formation of a particular judgment in regard to action. This interpretation is not new; it is defended also by Joannes a St. Thoma.[29] Fabro declares that in the process of perception the *eogitatativa* has the principal part, and is ultimately rooted in the intellect and not in the memory." This statement is not without some difficulty. How can a sensory faculty be "rooted" in the intellect? Every faculty, of course, *radicaliter oritur ex anima;* but this does not amount to the same. Insofar their relation to the soul is concerned, all faculties are rooted therein, as *accidentia propria.* It is also generally assumed that the sensory faculties, especially the external senses, are rooted in the *sensus communis* insofar it is this sense to which the process of sensory cognition devolves, the external senses only supplying, as it were, a still unformed material. (One is always reminded, when dealing with these questions, of Kant's notion of a "chaos of sensations" which is given significance only by the *a-priori* forms of *Anschauung.* This connection, conscious or not, of Kant's transcendental aesthetics with Aristotelean-Thomistic psychology explains somewhat why and how this epistemology could develop into a psychologistic interpretation with J. Fries, with H. v Helmholtz, in recent times with Sir Arthur Eddington.) It is not as easy to imagine a sensory function being rooted in a rational faculty.

One might be tempted to think that the relation between the soul and the body is somehow repeated or mirrored also in the relations obtaining between the single faculties. The being *propter intellectivum et non e converso* of the senses seems to correspond to the soul's being the final cause in the body. It may be permissible to say that the intellect is the final cause of the senses, or that the intellectual operations are the final cause of the performances of the sensory faculties. But

28 *Loc. cit.*

29 Joannes a St. Thoma, *Cursus philosophicus,* ed. Reiser, Taurin., 1937, III, 242, h. 32. (*Phil. nat.,* IV, q. 8, a. 1.) (*Aestimativa*) *in homine dicitur cogitativa quia cum aliqua collatione et discursu cogitat ei format intentiones, eo quod intentiones ex coniunctione ad intellectum modum quemdam discursivum participant.* This author credits the *vis cogitativa* with the capacity of apprehending other relations besides those of usefulness, etc., since he mentions among its objects also the relation of kinship, *ibid.,* a, 4 (p. 265, b. 21).

this does not as yet allow to speak *of* the latter being rooted in the former.

Whenever one has to deal with a hierarchical structure, great care is needed in analyzing the mutual relations between the strata of this hierarchy. The lower are generally a condition for the existence of the higher (within the created world); the latter are thus founded on the former, and depend also for their functioning and existence on them. The lower become subservient to the higher, since they have to supply to them a basis of existence and a substratum whereupon to exercise their power. The higher dominate the lower strata by subjecting them to themselves and making them, as it were, 'work in a manner suitable for the higher performances. These relations are often overlooked and confused, especially in modern psychology, because of the prevailing of some evolutionary idea which emphasizes exclusively the "development" of the higher "out" of the lower. Any evolutionary conception, of course, ends with abolishing the true notion of hierarchy, because this notion is incompatible with the other of continuity and gradual transformation underlying the evolutionary conception. The notion of "root" has to be interpreted according to similar viewpoints. It is not possible to use this notion without indicating in what particular sense one uses it.

Terms like being rooted, continuation, participation and others, veil more the difficulties than they contribute towards their solution. The problem, probably, can not be solved on the terrain of psychology alone. If we are to maintain the principle of distinguishing the faculties by their operations and their objects, we shall have to start further investigations from two sides: psychology has to find out more on and to give more detailed descriptions of the performances of the mind; ontology will have to investigate the nature of such objects as relation, situation, value. Only by a cooperation of the two sciences, any progress can be achieved.

That we are very much in need of a clearer knowledge of the objects mentioned just before, becomes clear when one considers another difficulty related to the problem of the *vis cogitativa*. It seems that this side of the problem has not aroused much attention in more recent times, but it was seen perfectly by older writers, for instance by Joannes a St. Thoma.[30] By what sensible data is the *vis cogitativa*

30 Joannes a St. Thoma, *Cursus Philosophicus*, ed. Reiser, Taurin., 1937, III, p. 265b. ff. (*Phil. Nat.*, IV, q. 8, a. 4.)

made cognizant of the *species insensatae*? What data allow this power to become aware, e.g. of the relation of usefulness, or of any other relation?

Many things, very different in nature and aspect, are useful or dangerous; many things are, in one sense or the other, goods. Even if one admits that "being good" is equivalent to "being good for me," the question still remains, on what sense-data this awareness rests. If values have no objective existence, are not even, as some have called them, "tertiary qualities," how does any act of appreciation arise at all? There is no help in referring to the phantasms as the way by which the res extra reaches the *vis cogitativa*. Any sense, it would seem, needs some kind of *species impressa* to be actualized. But if there is nothing objective in the object by 'which the sense may be impressed, no knowledge can ever arise. This problem becomes particularly hard to solve, when the object is supposed to be a relation obtaining between a *res extra* and the subject himself, as in the case of "dangerous for me." Joannes a St. Thoma was aware of these difficulties to which in fact he devotes a lengthy discussion. The *intentiones insensatae*, he says, being of a higher order require higher species or, at least, that the species be presented in a higher mode. There has to be some power or some agent generating these species more perfect than their origin out of the *sensa;* but it is impossible that the less perfect gives birth to the more perfect. The author, therefore concludes that these species are gained from the *sensa* themselves, since the latter "somehow contain" the former.

But this is not much of a solution; it is rather begging the question. Unless "being contained," is given a more definite explanation, we can not have any idea how the imperfect generates the perfect, or how the mind, is made aware of these *intentiones insensatae*. Joannes a St. Thoma apparently considers some process analogous to the abstraction of the universal nature from the phantasm. But, then, the universal nature is really present in the individual; it is not formed out of the less perfect, it is only disengaged from it. If this analogy is supposed to bold, one has to conclude that also what corresponds to the *species insensatae* is not only *tamquam* contained in the objects and therefore not only *iamquam* presented to the *vis cogitativa, but realitcr* present together with the other apprehendable characteristics and *realiter* distinct from them. That is, one arrives, with a certain inevitability, at an objectivistic conception of values.

It is quite true that there is a capacity of creation, *modo combinationis et divisionis,* also in the sensory faculties, especially in the *sensus communis* and in imagination. But this capacity can never explain the arising of something qualitatively new. Values are, by their nature, different from other intentional objects. To call them "subjective" or the result of an "objectivation " of "merely subjective" phenomena, to make them dependent of emotions or interests, etc. is no explanation at all. Such assertions are, in truth, only restatements of the original questions in a more veiled manner and in a less intelligible, though apparently more "scientific," language.

II

The actual state of the question shows that its ontological aspect has not as yet been clarified sufficiently to allow for any conclusive answer. One may ask whether there are not certain facts available which may prove helpful. Facts as such, of course, do not answer questions in ontology or speculation. But they may point a way towards a solution, provided they be true facts. This restriction, though obvious, is not always sufficiently considered. Philosophers easily take for facts what the authors in the various fields of empirical research declare to be such. The naked findings of the empiricist are not what he presents to us as a fact. He necessarily dads the findings into the language of his general conception. The "facts" are findings stated in a definite terminology. It is a finding, or an observation, that a stone deprived of support will fall to earth. It is a theory which states this observation by saying that the stone is "attracted" by the earth, or else that it seeks its natural place. It is an observation that animals behave under certain conditions regularly in a certain manner and that their behavior brings about certain effects; but it is a theory to assert that in animals "exist" instincts. An instinct is never observed; it is a notion introduced for the sake of having a common denominator for certain types of animal behavior.

But the empiricist as well as the philosopher who uses the former's statements are liable to overlook, the one by habit, the other by a sometimes not fully justified trust, the rôle played by the theoretical element in apparently purely descriptive statements. This is true also in regard to the problems with which these pages are occupied.

Referring to certain experiments on value-apprehension by W. Gruehn – of which more will be said presently – the learned author of one of the best known textbooks writes: "If Gruehn assumes the existence of an elementary form of consciousness apart from feeling and volition, it seems that this rests on an unduly narrow notion of feeling, which notion includes only sensual pleasantness and unpleasantness. But the phenomenon fits quite well into the series of higher feelings."[31] This statement evidently supposes that there can be no "elementary" form of consciousness besides those recognized by the author and many other psychologists. There is, however, no necessity at all to restrict the number of the elementary states. But a short time ago, the psychologists were compelled to acknowledge the existence of a peculiar state of consciousness they had overlooked until then and which to acknowledge they were indeed rather unwilling. But "thoughts" proved to be phenomena *sui generis*, not reducible to images and their combinations. It may be the same in case of value-apprehension.

It is not without a definite importance to the philosophy of the human mind whether values are apprehended by an operation sui generis or not. The faculties are, as has been pointed out before, distinguished by their operations and their objects. If we have sufficient reasons for assuming an operation distinct from those referring to other objects, we may-perhaps not conclude but-suspect that these objects too form a class of their own.

The experimental study of value-apprehension has been neglected more than the importance of the problem justifies. Few reliable studies exist which envision this problem. The reasons for this development can not be detailed here; they have little to do with the stand of experimental methods and. the development of psychology, and much with philosophical prejudices alive in the minds of the most "unphilosophical" students of mental phenomena. The more unphilosophical a mind is, the greater in number and influence are this mind's philosophical prejudices. No science can be more sure than the metaphysics is which it unconsciously and tacitly implies, as Prof. A. N. Whitehead justly remarked.

Among the few experimental studies on the psychology of value-apprehension the work of W. Gruehn deserves to be named in first place. It is looked at askance, of course, by those who believe only in figures.

31 J. Froebes, *Lehrbuch de experimentellen Psychologie*, 3d. ed., Freiburg i. B., 1929, Vol. II, p. 284.

There are neither correlation-tables nor tracings of curbs in Gruehn's book. It is, in spite of these "defects," a piece of serious and of effective research.[32]

The following brief description on how the mind becomes aware of values and proceeds to appreciate them, to assuming a definite attitude in regard of them, is based mostly on Gruehn's researches, partly however on observations made and ideas developed by the present writer.

Gruehn is a pupil of Girgensohn's whose great work on *The Psychology of Religious Experience* he re-edited. He is a Protestant theologian, well versed in experimental psychology. The method adopted by him is the one called "experimental self-observation," developed first by O. Kuelpe and his school. His observers were mostly students of theology. Their statements proved to be valuable, because of their personal interest in the problem, and because of the previous training to which they had been subjected. The descriptions of the evaluating process as given by the various observers show a remarkable uniformity in the main features.

Two of them deserve particular attention. It became evident that an evaluation, i.e. an awareness of value and of its rank, may exist without a corresponding feeling-state or even together with one opposite to the kind of value. It is, of course, true that the awareness of a positive value is generally accompanied by a feeling of pleasure. But it is not true that such an awareness depends on a pleasant feeling as a necessary condition. This fact can be ascertained also by common observation, under average, non-experimental conditions. But, so far as attention has been paid to this fact, it has been listed among the many "self-deceptions," a name commonly given to all mental facts not fitting into some preconceived theory. It is not difficult at all to bring together many observations which show that emotions-or feelings-appear as responses to the awareness of values, but that the latter state may be present and its object recognized without the intervention of any feeling. The manyfold theories which conceive of values as "merely subjective" and which refer to the emotions, doubtless subjective states, as the basis of our value-awareness rest on insufficient observations, or rather on an arbitrary neglect of certain facts, deemed to be unimportant, illusionary, or what not.

The second important feature of evaluation discovered by Gruehn is what he calls the "act of appropriation" (respectively of rejection).

32 W. Gruehn, *Der Werterlebnis*, Leipzig, 1924.

A value may be recognized as such and even be given its place within some scale of values, and nevertheless "leave one cold." Unless this value becomes, as it were, incorporated in the person's moral or aesthetic attitudes, it remains outside, merely existent, without any reference to the self. There is in processes of evaluation a definite step by which the purely observational attitude changes into one corresponding the *tua res agitur*. This also is the moment in which an emotional response sets in. True, the emotional response often appears as co-instantaneous with the awareness of the object. But this results from the fact that many evaluations have become habitual and also that there are certain values – perhaps this is more frequently the case with disvalues – which are common to all men.

This act of appropriation is held by Gruehn to be a mental phenomenon of a peculiar nature, not reducible to others, experienced as clearly distinct from feelings – even higher ones – and constituting the very essence of true evaluation. In spite of Froebes' criticism, the existence and the peculiarity of this phenomenon seems to be sure. We then have to consider this act of appropriation as an "elementary" phenomena. If it is such one, it demands a special mental activity, and underlying this activity, a special faculty.

There are, of course, numerous studies which emphasize the rôle of emotions in the process of value-awareness. Since it is not the intention of the present writer to give a complete report on the literature, these studies need not be considered. But it is worthy of notice that Gruehn is, by far, not the only author who speaks of a non-emotional awareness of -values. Among the philosophers who deal with the question mention has to be made of D. v. Hildebrand who rejects the idea of emotions being the basis of our evaluations and of our knowledge of values."[33] O. Stapledon holds a similar view.[34] Recently E. Eller has stressed the point that value-awareness is of the nature of cognition and not of feeling. To this author, the fact of temptation is a conclusive demonstration of the objectivity of vaines. "If man would procreate out of himself the world of

33 D. v. Hildebrand, "Die Idee der sittlichen Handlung," *Jahrb. f. Phaenomenol.*, 1930, III.

34 O. Stapledon, "The Bearing of Ethics on Psychology," *Journ. Phil.*, 1927, II, 373.

vaines, he never would permit such a painful to and fro to arise as it is conditioned by temptation.[35]

G. F. Moore has pointed out a fact, indeed of common observation, but usually neglected by the empirical psychologists. He says: "Not only is the pleasantness of a state not in proportion to its intrinsic worth; it may even add positively to its vileness."[36] But it is hardly possible to have two contradicting feelings coexist in one's mind. If value depended on feeling, the situation alluded to by Moore hardly even would arise. It is also quite true that "it will always remain pertinent to ask, whether the feeling itself is good."[37] And if this is the case, the emotional theory of values would necessitate a second feeling by which the value of the first, allegedly determining the value awareness, becomes known to the mind. Thus an infinite regress would result.

B. M. Laing too refers to the fact that it is the value as apprehended which arouses desire, and not desire on which value is founded.[38] The disagreement between emotion and the known worth of a thing or action is emphasized also by L. R. Ward.[39] Most clearly the dependence of emotions on values previously cognized is pointed out by J. Laird, who also refers to the incompatibility of contradictory emotions while it is quite possible that the same fact may be apprehended in its different aspects both as a value and a disvalue. "Sympathetic pain ... may be a disvalue *qua* pain, and, a value *qua* sympathetic."[40] If, however the disvalue of pain were transmitted to the mind by a feeling of unpleasantness, and the value by a pleasurable feeling, such a situation could not exist at all.

The psychologist Th. Ribot states that in value-awareness there is, besides an emotional factor one which he describes as "resembling to the purely intellectual concept."[41] M. E. Clarke, though

35 E. Eller, "Die Versuchung in wertphilosophischer Sicht," *Stimm. d. Zeit,* 1939, CXXXVII, 26.

36 G.E. Moore, *Principia Ethica,* Cambridge, 1922, p. 214.

37 *Ibid.,* p. 41.

38 B. M. Laing, "On Value," *Philos.,* 1935, X, 44.

39 L. R. Ward, Philosophy of Value, New York, 1930, p. 135. (Also Cath. Univ. Diss., Washington, D.C., 1939.)

40 J. Laird, *The Idea of Value,* Cambridge, 1929, p. 351.

41 Th. Ribot, *La logique des sentiments,* 3d ed., Paris, 1920, p. 36.

doubting whether there is any example of value-awareness devoid of emotional elements, declares that in such phenomena enters a non-intellectual apprehension of value which is not cognition "in the ordinary sense ... for it is not an intellectual matter."[42] The author does, however, not draw the obvious conclusion that the facts she refers to necessitate the assumption of a non-intellectual and nevertheless cognitive faculty.

No words, perhaps, summarize the state of things better than a remark of St. Thomas does, when be writes that a thing is enjoyed for it own sake and not only because of the effect on us.[43] The good is, he says elsewhere,[44] that which first falls *into the apprehension of the practical reason. This reason, even if it is taken to be* an aspect of the intellect, can not operate unless it *be* referred to the particular thing or action. The apprehension of the particular *bonum* has to be entrusted to a faculty capable of getting in touch with the particular.

It is characteristic of the dominating spirit in recent psychology that the items value, evaluation, and such like are absent from practically all treatises. Correlated to this blindness for certain facts regarding values is the unwillingness of modern psychologists to acknowledge the existence of will as a particular mental phenomenon. But no one can deny that decision, purpose, volition exist as well defined experiences everyone has of his one mind. If psychology pretends that there is no will, it has to explain how and why this general belief arose. Little is done by referring to the influence of names and declaring that the "substantivation" makes man's belief in the existence as a "thing" of anything which has a name. Little is done with this, because then the question has to be asked why some nothing has come to be considered as a thing. All these so-called explanations amount only to shifting the question to another level, and never are any kind of answer. It is the same with values. Declaring then to be "merely subjective" and attributed to reality only by some error of tb mind or by some habit of the mind, has no explanatory worth. Values are experienced; they are sides of reality not less than any other qualities are. If all qualities are

42 M. E. Clarke, "Cognition and Affection in the Experience of Value," *Jour. Phil.*, 1938, XXXV, 5.

43 *Summa Theol.*, II-II, q. 7, a. 1c.

44 *Summa Theol.*, I-II, q. 94, a. 2c.

said to be "subjective," nothing is gained, because the question remains the sane within subjectivity.

Now, if there is a mental operation *sui generic* by which we become aware of values, then the presumption becomes more plausible that there are particular objects corresponding to this operation and a particular faculty underlying them.

Gruehn, when reporting on his experimental studies, was not interested in such problems, nor did he think in terms of Thomistic psychology. The existence or non-existence of some faculty was nothing he might have considered. Nor did be, probably, know of the notion of the *vis cogitativa*. But his statements seem to be in perfect accordance with what one might expect on the basis of this notion.

The findings of the psychologist, therefore, are rather suggestive. If it is true that the task of the *vis cogitativa*, according to St. Thomas, or at least to his principles, is not limited to the apprehension of the useful or the dangerous and of eventually some few other relations between on objective datum and the person, but extends to the awareness of any particular value, realized or capable of realization in a particular object, or situation, then it well seems that the discovery of this act of appropriation may be considered a proof for the operation of this internal sense.

Many questions, of greater or lesser importance, are closely related to these things. It has been pointed out already that there are some problems awaiting clarification. Much work has to be done until the philosophical and the empirical approach to the problems of the mind will be brought together and be made to co-operate effectively. But it seems not without some importance that one be made aware of a certain parallelism between the questions arising in both fields. The situations in present philosophy and in present psychology point in the same direction. The gap between these two endeavors of man for understanding reality and himself apparently may become less wide. Some kind of bridge may be thrown over. Mutual understanding is the necessary condition for co-operation. But no co-operation can ever be brought about so long as the philosopher ignores the doings of the psychologist, and the latter thinks unimportant what the former says.

THE COGNITIVE ASPECT OF EMOTIONS

Traditional psychology considers emotional states as the conscious reflexes, so to speak, of the movements of the sensory appetites. Whenever a value embodied in some particular is apprehended by the cogitative power (*vis cogitativa*) and a correspondent movement of the appetite ensues, there is in the consciousness one of the passions of the soul (*passiones animae*), varying according to the objective relation between the good and the person. It has, perhaps, been too little emphasized that this psychology takes into account, not only the subjective side, but also the total situation in which the person is involved. In this sense, Thomistic psychology is very "modern." It is only recently that psychology has discovered this dependence of mental states and total behavior sets on the general situation.

In traditional psychology, the apprehension of the moving agent, the good or the evil, as embodied in some object, is achieved by the fourth internal sense, the cogitative power (*vis cogitativa*).[1] The cognition of the goodness or badness of the object, event, or situation, precedes the movement of the appetite and, therefore, the consciousness of an emotional state. Thus far, the old conception agrees with certain recent theories. If, however, these theories conceive of the emotions as a mere mirroring of a biologically relevant set of circumstances or even – as did the famous James-Langi-Sergi theory – consider emotions as the awareness of bodily changes, wrought by biological forces released in their turn by the environmental circumstances, Scholastic tradition disagrees. A mental cognitive factor has to enter into play. For the appetites, and their emotional effects too, the proposition is valid that nothing can be willed but what is previously known. Replace "willed" by "sought" and the statement applies to the appetites not less than to rational will.

1 R. Allers, "The *Vis Cogitativa* and Evaluation," *The New Scholasticism*, XV (1941), p. 195.

There is a great divergence of opinions regarding the nature and definition of emotions. The Wittenberg Symposium Feelings and Emotions, of 1928, lists as many definitions as there are contributors. And things have not changed since then. It seems, therefore, advisable to summarize briefly the conception of emotion underlying the present discussion.

An emotion is a mental state of peculiar character by which an individual responds to the awareness of a pleasant or unpleasant situation, or any other aspect of a situation entailing goodness or badness. This response is of the whole individual, mental and bodily, not of the mind or of consciousness alone.

Emotion, therefore, presupposes the awareness of the value-aspect of a situation. This awareness may be purely sensory apprehension such as is found also in animals and credited, by traditional psychology, to the *vis aestimativa*, one of the internal senses. Such a mere sensory awareness may occur also with man. Usually, however, the value awareness is, in man, of a higher order, namely an intellectual apprehension, founded on the sensory awareness of a particular value as embodied in the actually present situation.

The bodily alterations associated with emotion become partly conscious and color the emotional consciousness. Emotion may be described as the consciousness of a change "affecting" the whole human person. It refers to objects as causes, not in the way of cognition nor in the way of appetition.

Contrary to some modern notions, traditional psychology does not credit emotion with any cognitive power. Nor is it the foundation of evaluation. Neither "interest" nor "pleasure" constitutes the awareness of value or goodness. A thing is of "interest" because it is good, or bad; it does not become good or bad because the person is interested. The philosophy of values, as conceived by R. B. Perry,[2] is as much a reversal of the true state of things, as James' theory is such a reversal in regard to the relation between emotion and bodily changes. Professor Perry has remained true to the spirit of his master.

The only thing which is indubitably true is that there obtains a close relation between the awareness of values and emotional states. This relation has been interpreted in a new manner by two authors. Max Scheler, in his *Der Formalismus in der Ethik und die materiale*

2 For a criticism of Perry's philosophy of values, cf. H. E. Cory, "Value, Beauty, and Professor Perry," *The Thomist*, IV (1942), 1.

Wertethik[3] has advocated a theory of emotional cognition of values. Alexius von Meinong has spoken of values as "dignitatives" and as being the proper object of a particular class of cognitive emotional states. Values are, according to this philosopher, "presented" to consciousness by means of emotional states.[4] It is not the intention of the present writer to enter into a detailed criticism of these two theories. Only a few objections, which apparently cannot be met by these conceptions, will be mentioned.

There is first the fact to which G. E. Moore has referred, that we evaluate not only objects but our feelings themselves. This remark has been directed mainly against those who make feeling states, of pleasantness or unpleasantness, the very basis of evaluation. But it applies no less to the theories of emotional value cognition. In both cases it leads to an infinite regress. Furthermore, it is inconceivable that a feeling state be felt by a feeling of second order.[5] Secondly, the testimony of simple consciousness is evidently opposed to the theory of emotional value cognition. Everyone, probably, knows of cases in which he is aware of a value, embodied in some particular object, and nonetheless does not react emotionally. We may perfectly see" the value of a painting, and nevertheless dislike it, not of course because we, e.g., disapprove of it as immoral or something similar, but because it "leaves us cold." Nor is it true that a value is recognized at one time and not recognized at another time, although our emotional reactions may present considerable differences. A symphony does not become less beautiful, even to our own mind, if it does not appeal to us in the mood in which we find ourselves at a particular time.

Also, the relation between emotions and values is shown by immediate consciousness as being of another kind than the cognitive relation between, say, a sense object and a perception, or an intellectual truth and a judgment. Language takes account of this difference. We see, perceive, think something, or we think "of" something. But we are sad because or about, angered by, ashamed because of, worried about, and so forth. Language is, of course, not always a reliable guide. But it

3 Halle a. S.: M. Niemeyer, 1916. Appeared first in Husserl's *Jahrbuch für Philosophie und phaemomenologische Forschung.*

4 "Uber emotionale Praesentation," *Sitz. Ber. Wiener Akad. d. Wissensch.* Phil. Kl. *1917.*

5 G. E. Moore, *Principia ethica.*

is, after all, the crystallization, as it were, of popular psychology and to a certain extent a witness for the general ideas of mankind.

Scheler emphasized very much the "objectivity" of values and credited therefore the "intentional feelings," of which he spoke, with a true cognitive capacity. It is doubtful whether such "intentional feelings" can be demonstrated at all. It seems to this writer as if there were always a separation possible, by introspective analysis, of the feeling, or emotional state, on one hand and the value awareness on the other. The main argument is, of course, the actual occurrence of the two states independently of each other.

While philosophers and psychologists in general were agreed that feelings are "merely subjective" and denote only a modification of the ego as a response to certain affections, a thinker who then was hardly noticed had developed, incidentally, a very different conception. This conception was worked out neither with a philosophical nor with a psychological intention. The man who had a novel interpretation of emotional states to offer was interested not in philosophical but in religious questions. But his was an uncanny capacity for psychological analysis, equalled only by a contemporary of his who in other things was his opposite. The one author is the Danish theologian Sören Kierkegaard; his opposite is Frederick Nietzsche.

Kierkegaard wanted to show what man can be at his best, when fully realizing his situation and surrendering to divine grace. Nietzsche wanted to "unveil" the depths of human nature and show man at his worst, although he too desired man to rise above his baseness. While Kierkegaard made man's rise dependent on the recognition of the essential finiteness of human nature, Nietzsche hoped that man would rise above himself by his own power. While the one proclaimed, with an earnestness not equalled, perhaps, since the times of the Fathers, man the creature of the infinite God, the other proudly exclaimed, "God is dead," and saw in all religion the expression of cowardice and resentment.

Sharpsighted though Nietzsche was and though he anticipated many of the psychological insights of later times, he nevertheless proved less able to gauge the depths of human nature than did Kierkegaard. Nietzsche's understanding of the mind was handicapped by his pronounced naturalistic attitude, his biologistic outlook, his enthusiasm for science and evolutionary ideas. Accordingly, he could not conceive of emotions otherwise than as biologically valuable phenomena, indicative of health or disease, strength or weakness, power or slavery. Nietzsche's ideas, therefore, may be left out of consideration in the present context.

Of the Kierkegaardian ideas, however, only those regarding emotional states have to be considered here. Kierkegaard was not, as has been remarked, primarily a psychologist. His penetrating analysis of emotions is merely one link of the chain of reasoning by which he endeavors to develop a philosophical anthropology, an idea of man based on philosophical principles indeed, but even more on revealed truth and on the testimony of conscience. Kierkegaard is introspective to the highest degree, and he is so with unusual success. His views have gained influence on writers who are far from sharing Kierkegaard's impassioned religiosity.

Two emotions received particular attention in Kierkegaard's works: dread and despair. On the first he wrote a separate treatise, The Concept of Dread, and the second is one of the fundamentals of his The Sickness unto Death.[6] These two works the author himself characterized as "psychological." The analysis of these two states which will be given below is largely indebted to Kierkegaard, but also to some authors who made dread an object of special study and who were dependent in many ways on the ideas of the Dane. It seems, therefore, unnecessary to report on Kierkegaard's views in detail.

Scientific psychology did not come under the influence of Kierkegaard or Nietzsche. Among those who were concerned not so much with the study of mental facts and operations, but with the mind itself or with human personality, some made their own consciously or unconsciously took over many of the ideas contained in the writings of Kierkegaard and Nietzsche. Psychoanalysis makes use of several notions and terms introduced by Nietzsche. Another current in psychopathology is largely fed from Kierkegaardian sources. Freud stated that he was not acquainted with any of Nietzsche's works when he conceived the basic notions of his system. The similarity, however, is too striking for mere coincidence. We have no reason to doubt Freud's statement. But, as this writer has pointed out elsewhere[7] there were many channels through which Nietzsche's ideas may have reached

6 *The Sickness unto Death,* trans. W. Lowrie. Princeton: Princeton University Press, 1941. *Der Begriff der Angst,* trans. Schrempf. Jena: E. Diederichs, 1912.

7 *The Successful Error,* New York, Sheed & Ward, 1940.

Freud and been taken over by him without his knowing whence these ideas came to him.

Not only psychopathologists and psychologists who were interested in questions scientific or experimental psychology could not and would not answer, but also philosophers came under the influence of both Nietzsche and Kierkegaard. The former's ideas spread over a wide field. They will not occupy us here. The latter's notions became effective especially in the philosophical work of Martin Heidegger.[8] Of this work only those parts will be considered which deal with the nature and significance of emotional states. Heidegger's most detailed analysis is of dread. Some remarks on other emotions occur incidentally.

Heidegger's philosophy is too complicated to be even sketched.[9] His interpretation of dread forms an integral part of the system, but this part may be detached from the whole and considered in the light of descriptive psychology. A brief summary of Heidegger's views on dread will enable us to put forth the corrections and enlargements this view seems to demand.

Heidegger emphasizes justly the difference between fear and dread, as Kierkegaard had done before. Fear, the German philosopher claims, is the response to something threatening (the term *das Abträgliche* would be best translated by "nocive") apprehended as coming from a definite direction which is known as is the threatening thing itself. It is approaching; it is not yet here, but is within a relatively close distance. Fear implies the possibility that the threat will not be realized. Since the thing feared is known, it belongs to the world in which man dwells.

Dread or anxiety is quite different. That which is dreaded is essentially the unknown, that "where we are not at home"; it is, as an expressive German word has it, *das Un-heimliche,* which term names exactly the general mood of strangeness, of uncanniness, which takes hold of

8 *Sein und Zeit,* Halle a. S.: Niemeyer, 1927. *Was ist Metaphysik?* Bonn: Cohen, 1929.

9 Heidegger is exceedingly difficult reading, even for one who is perfectly acquainted with the German language. The articles published by W. H. Cerf, "An Approach to Heidegger," and by W. H. Werkmeister, "An Introduction to Heidegger's Existential Philosophy," *Philosophy and Phenomenological Research, I* (1940), 177, and II (1941), 79, are helpful towards a first understanding.

the mind in an utterly new and unknown situation. As the dreaded something is unknown, so is the direction and the region from which it will strike. One may refer to the dread some experience when there is apparently nothing to be dreaded, e.g., in complete silence. *Ipsa quies rerum mundique silentia terrent* (Cf. Valerius Flaccus, *Argonautica*, II, 41). The well known dreadful property of complete darkness equally belongs here. Therefore, dread has an all-surrounding character. It is everywhere, there is no escaping, especially since the dreaded unknown, unknown though it be, is anticipated as inevitable. From somewhere it is sure to strike, and to strike with an annihilating power. It does not strike as yet, else we would cease to be, but it is not at any distance, it is immediately close to us. As an unknown it cannot be placed; nevertheless it is everywhere, surrounding us, bearing down on us, oppressing us. (Oppression is one of the most prominent characteristics of the experience of dread, which gives to this state its name in Greek, Latin, and German, the common root "*ang*" which refers to restriction or confinement in a too narrow space.)

Heidegger considers then two aspects of dread: the mind, or rather the person, dreads something and dreads because of something, that is, man is aware – although with a peculiar kind of awareness – of the threat and of the threatened.[10]

10 Heidegger's way of dealing with the German language is peculiar and quite often arbitrary. He gives new and unwonted significance to certain terms and coins new ones. Sometimes the use he makes of words throws an unexpected light on connotations which are usually overlooked. But sometimes also the reader can hardly help feeling that many of Heidegger's statements, ostensibly of ontological import, are in truth only gathered from language. This becomes manifest whenever one tries to render Heidegger's ideas in another language than German. Then statements he presents as evident become more than questionable. Werkmeiester, in the article mentioned in note (9), expresses similar views.

One is tempted to ask why and how a philosopher of undoubted capacity, passionately interested in the problems of being, should rely so much on evidence as peripherical as meanings of words are. This may be partly explained by remembering that Heidegger is a pupil of Husserl. The latter believes that to every mode of experience belongs and corresponds a mode of being, at least in the sense of *esse intentionale*. What the ultimate ontological conception of Husserl may have been is not a problem of the present discussion.

The other root, which may be assumed with good reason, is to be discovered in Heidegger's own development and work. One of his earliest writings,

That which is threatened and that for which man, when in dread, trembles is, according to Heidegger, the "being in the-world." This being in the world is to this philosopher the very mode of being, the existence of man is being in the world. This particular interpretation will not be questioned for the moment. It is, however, necessary to inquire into the justness of the phenomenological or descriptive analysis.

It is true that dread puts before the person the possibility of annihilation. This annihilation, contrary to what Heidegger seems to imply, is not the loss of being in the world, but the loss of value. This becomes clear if one surveys the modifications of dread. All of them have in common the feature of an imminent "fall." Dread dreads the fall from a value level held or attained to one much lower, finally down to the

---

in fact the one by which he received the *venia legendi* in philosophy, deals with language. The title is *Die Kategorien und Bedeutungslehre des Duns Scotus* (Tübingen Mohr, 1916). Its topic is an analysis of the *Grammatica Speculativa*, a treatise which figures among the writings of Duns Scotus, but whose author is, as M. Grabmann was able to show, Thomas of Erfurt (Thomas Erfordiae) of the fourteenth century (Grabmann, *Mittelalterliches Geistesleben*, Vol. I. Munich: M. Hueber, 1926). Incidentally, Grabmann mentions a fact which may serve as an explanation for the mistaken attribution. Thomas was rector in a convent *apud Scotus* at Erfurt, and thus himself became Scotus. The famous author curiously has overlooked this connection.

The treatises *De Grammatica Speculativa* or *De Modis Significandi* contain usually a reference to a strict correspondence between modes of being, of understanding, and of signifying. This idea is maintained even by authors who, by their adherence to nominalism and, accordingly, to the view that words are arbitrary signs (*signa ad placitum*) – while concepts are natural signs (*signa natura1ia*) – ought to abandon the strict correspondence between concepts or their modes, and words.

Heidegger's rather striking tendency to treat an ambiguity in words as if it necessarily referred to a two sided ontological fact, and his whole habit of making much out of idioms and peculiarities of language, may be traced back to the ideas with which he became imbued when studying the treatise of Thomas Erfordiae. This is the more probable since throughout the work dealing with "Scotus" he attempts to modernize the medieval notions as much as possible. He discovers striking similarities between the views of the medieval author and certain modern, particularly Husserlian, ideas. Thus, the melting into one of his fundamental philosophical intuitions with the conception of the modistae, seems a not improbable explanation.

absolute non value which, of course, is also the level of non existence. *Ens et bonum, convertuntur.*[11]

Heidegger has a very peculiar concept of *das Nichts,* the Nought. It is nothing and nevertheless is powerful enough to threaten with annihilation. There is indubitably a relation of dread and Nought. But it appears to this writer in a manner rather different from Heidegger's interpretation. The Nought is not, as Heidegger believes, that which threatens with annihilation, but that whereto man is driven by a power infinitely superior to his own, and where annihilation awaits him. Dread makes us feel "powerless." But such a notion is meaningless in face of the Nought; it has a meaning only if we are faced by some power superior to our own. The Nought is not that which threatens but rather that – if such an expression be permitted – whereto we are threatened. Dread reveals to man his nothingness.

Heidegger has not quite overlooked this, inasmuch as he declares that in dread man is faced by his finitude. But finitude without an infinite gives no sense. The infinite is, *nautra rei,* the primary; the finite is only because of and in regard to the infinite; it is secondary. That the infinite is "discovered" only by starting from the finite does not make any difference. We know of many instances in which that which is prior in nature (*natura*) is secondary in our knowledge (*quoad nos*). Nor should we be disturbed by the verbal form of negation. Language repeatedly has a negative name for what is actually the positive. "Innocence "is one of the most striking examples.

Man in understanding himself as finite grasps at the same time, however vaguely and inadequately, the infinite. The infinite is what threatens with annihilation. Being in its fullness, the *ὄντος ὄν,* confronts finite and contingent being with the necessity of realizing its finiteness and contingency.

By this one also understands the close relation obtaining between dread and the attitude of revolt. The finite being, made aware of its finiteness, revolts and asserts itself in a *non serviam.* (Here may be found also the reasons for the dread and the unruly pride or ambition which are at the bottom of so called neurotic troubles. Kierkegaard

11 This and many of the following remarks summarize briefly a more detailed study the present writer published years ago. "Zur Phaenomenologie und Metaphysik der Angst," *Religion und Seelenleben,* VII (1932) 157 165. (Proc. of the Section of Psychology, Deutscher Kathol. Akademikerverband.)

has seen something of this, although he was not primarily interested in psychopathology.)

Dread, then, discloses to the person experiencing this emotion something of his, or of man's, nature. This "knowledge," if it deserves to be called so in its initial stages, becomes true knowledge only in reflection. Reflection, however, is not possible while dread lasts, since this emotion paralyzes all activities. The awareness of finitude is none the less effective; even while dread lasts man is conscious, only in an implicit and unreflected manner, of his contingency and finitude. One wonders whether something of this sort is adumbrated in the words: "The fear of the Lord is the beginning of wisdom."

The awareness of finitude and contingency, that is, of the nature of a created being, explains also the close relations obtaining between dread and the sentiment of guilt. Anxiety of conscience is, in its pure cases, not simply fear of punishment. Servile fear, says St. Bernard, is the lowest degree of obedience. Such an anxiety may arise irrespective of all ideas of punishment, just as a good action may be achieved irrespective of all reward. The good conscience does not imply any idea of future reward; good is not done for the sake of being a deserving one (*bene meritus*), but for the sake of the right and good itself. It is the most perfect exercise of freedom, which St. Anselm defined as "rightness sought for itself" (*rectitudo propter se servata*). The knowledge of having failed to preserve this rightness and thus having failed to maintain one's position in regard to the order of goodness brings about the sentiment of guilt, just as the awareness of one's failing to acknowledge the position in regard to the order of being is at the bottom of dread. Dread indeed may cease to exist, or even may cease to be possible, when man fully realizes his being as contingent, finite, dependent, and maintained in existence by the infinite power and being Himself. *Superba anima formidinis ancilla,* as St. Johannes Climacus has it. (It is, incidentally, not uninteresting to note that among the several pseudonyms Kierkegaard used, also figures the one of Climacus.) However, it may be doubtful whether freedom from dread can be achieved in this life. The full realization and acceptance of what it means to be a creature can be had, perhaps, only in "seeing [God] face to face."

Kierkegaard has written extensively, in *The Sickness unto Death,* on a state, one can hardly say of mind, rather of the human person, which he calls "despair." In fact, the word he uses has no equivalent in English nor in any other language besides those of the German family.[12]

It is doubtful whether despair as conceived by Kierkegaard may be referred to as an emotion, because this despair is a state of things essentially hidden to consciousness. Man is in a state of despair, but he does not know it. This despair exists in two forms: "desperately wanting to be oneself" and "desperately wanting to be not oneself." In both cases, it seems, this despair is of the nature of a revolt. He who desperately wants to be himself desires to make himself the absolute. This was Nietzsche's kind of despair – " If there were God, how could I support not being God myself." Therefore, "God is dead." But he who desires, with equal desperation, not to be himself, who desires as it were to become transformed into another, is also in revolt against his given – by Fate or by God, according as he sees it – person. He wants to be more by becoming another. Both enterprises are condemned to fail. They cannot even be started, unless in an imaginary and fictitious way. (Here too, the relation to problems of the psychology of neurosis is apparent.) An impossible enterprise, one bound to fail, one whose failure can be foreseen with absolute certainty, may condition a state of despair. We say, "I despair of ever reaching this or that goal," because we are conscious of the impossibility.

Now, what Kierkegaard calls despair is apparently not the emotion itself but a mode of this senseless craving to get rid of oneself, existentially, in becoming another, or, essentially, by being thoroughly

---

12 It is not without interest to observe the expressions used by various languages for such a fundamental fact as despair. Latin, of course, is the source for the English and the French word, also that of the Italian or any other Romance language. The Greek has several terms, one which simply means "loss of hope," but two others which perhaps are particularly characteristic of the Greek mentality. They refer indeed to the incapacity of understanding (ἀπονοεἰσθαι), or the insolubility of the situation (ἀπορεῖν). The German term, however, is *Verzweifelung*, which implies the notion of two (*zwei*) and of doubt (*Zweifel*), and thus indicates that in despair there is no solution possible, that all doubting in regard to the outcome is over, that the terrible event or state has become irrevocably real. That this is one aspect of despair did not escape Aquinas, who says that desperation, exceeding the measure of fear (*mensura timoris*), sets in when there is no chance of any change taking place. But popular psychology, or the prevailing mentality of s people, evidently has felt one feature more characteristic there and another elsewhere.

and exclusively oneself, that is, independently so. The author uses the formula, "desperately wanting," thus indicating that despair is something inherent in this nonsensical endeavor. But this formula leaves the question open whether or not true despair may be found also outside of the situation envisioned by Kierkegaard. He seems to imply that despair and this craving are really distinct, although perhaps they are not separable in the sense that despair exists independently of this craving. It might be that only the craving gives rise to a state of true despair, but it might also be that despair can be attached, as it were, to other situations.

To answer this question a very thorough analysis of despair, real and alleged, is necessary, an undertaking which cannot be started here. One thing, however, seems to be sure. Despair is the response of the person to a final situation entailing a great evil. This is also the meaning Aquinas gives to *desperatio*. Despair, then, is another form in which man becomes aware of and is faced by the absoluteness of his finitude. The aspect of finitude as revealed in despair is different from the one revealed in dread, or anxiety of conscience. These two latter states reveal to man his status within the realm of being and of value. Despair teaches him – or it might teach him, if he did not, as Kierkegaard indicates, manage by some trick to remain unaware of his own desperate state – the limitation of his power. In the two forms of Kierkegaardian despair there is visible the catastrophe and final defeat of the "will of power," the central idea of Nietzsche. Long before man can have evolved, as Nietzsche hoped he would, to a superhuman state, he falls prey to despair.

The "origin" of dread has been placed, by authors who hold a more biological view, in the fact of death and of all those situations which, consciously understood or not, are premonitory of the finitude of life. But it seems more in accordance with facts to say that the dread of death (the usual term, "fear of death," ought to be discarded because death is essentially unknown) is but one instance of the general dread related to the revelation of finitude. That life ends is only one side of this finitude.

Human finitude presents a threefold aspect. It is finitude of being, and to its revelation corresponds the emotion of dread, and on a less deep level the emotion of fear, since the frightful situation has the note of threat in common with the dreadful situation. Finitude is, secondly, the limitation of the realization of the ideal, be it a true or a false one.

Man is condemned to remain always far below that which he wishes to be. Of course, there are many, too many, who never admit to themselves, much less to others, that they are far from what they want or at least once wanted to be. If they still admit their previous ideals, they are apt to talk of them smilingly, in a half pitying way, deriding the foolishness of youthful ideas, and emphasizing how much wiser, how much more sensible, more aware of "what life really is" they have become. These are the people who, according to Kierkegaard, are in a state of despair without knowing about this state. Were they to become conscious of their actual state, they would have made the first step beyond it, just as contrition is the step by which man elevates himself, helped indeed by divine grace, above the level on which to commit the sin was "natural" to him. Despair is the emotion corresponding to the finitude which is evident in the distance between the ideal view and the real being of man. If one is willing to make a concession to the terminology adopted by some, one may say that dread is related to the finitude of existence and despair to the finitude of essence. Man, however, is not only impotent to realize himself, to become fully himself, that is, to actualize all his potentialities, but also is incapable of realizing his purposes in the world without. The greatest achievements, even if for the moment they gave intense satisfaction to their creator, are inevitably below what inspiration and expectation depicted to his mind. The incapacity to deal with the objective world as he would like to do reveals to man another aspect of his finitude, one by which he is made aware that he is not able to form the world, not even of the infrahuman beings, according to his desires. There is resistance of matter, of things and persons; there are material and temporal conditions independent of man's will.

These experiences, innumerable and of divers impressiveness, make evident to man not only his lack of power, the fact that he is far from almightiness, much though he may dream of it, but also assure him that he belongs to the world. No experience is so much able to refute the theoretical (although never practical) solipsism than the resistance encountered on the part of others. And nothing gives so much right to a realistic interpretation of "being in the world" than the fact of the stubbornness and unmalleability of material things. The importance of the experience of resistance for the justification of realism has been emphasized by several thinkers in recent times (e.g., N. Hartmann).

"Being in the world" means also "being with others" (*Mitsein*, as Heidegger says). Thus, it overcomes the loneliness of the individual, sometimes so much that the individual person ceases to be wholly himself and gets lost, engulfed by the "many." (Incidentally it may be noted that in this point not only is Heidegger definitely indebted to Kierkegaard, but there is also a curious similarity in the ideas of Kierkegaard-Heidegger on the one hand, and Nietzsche on the other. One recalls the latter's word of the "too many." Heidegger, for that matter, is not altogether independent of Nietzsche either.)

In this aspect of human finitude there is a feature which Kierkegaard might have called a "dialectical" reversal. The very fact which, envisioned from one side, depresses man by revealing his finitude, gives to him, seen from another side, a security he never would call his own were he perfectly isolated. It is on the level of this awareness – which, however, need not be and usually is not explicitly realized – that communion with others develops.

It is one of the most striking features in Heidegger's philosophy that he so much dwells on the tragic, or at least uncomfortable, sides of human existence, and that he has no word either on love or pity or any of the "*Sympathiegefühle*" to which Scheler has devoted so much attention and on which he has shed so much light.[13] But if it is true that emotional states have, whatever their role may be besides, the function of revealing to man, in a peculiar manner, something of his position in the order of being, his "ontic status," and, accordingly, of his nature, it would be exceedingly improbable that only the negative emotions, like dread or despair, should be gifted with such a power.

Generally speaking, it seems that these negative emotions hinder objective knowledge more than the positive emotional states do. There is, of course, a blindness for facts born of optimism. But the distortion of objectivity wrought by pessimism usually goes much farther. It is not only because he has greater courage and a more hopeful outlook that the optimist generally achieves more than the pessimist. History seems to teach that the pessimists never achieved anything truly noticeable. It is also, and perhaps chiefly, because the optimist, as long as he still uses his reason, has a truer conception of reality.

The emotional reaction released by the awareness of the insurmountable resistance offered by reality is obviously anger. This is in accordance with the notion that the *malum arduum* is the adequate

13 *Wesen und Formen der Sympathiegefühle*, 2d ed. Bonn: Cohen, 1923.

object of the irascible appetite and conditions anger. Although this emotion may sometimes set free unexpected forces in the person, it is mostly impotent anger, especially since many facts which make us angry belong to the past. That this or that occurred, was done, by oneself or by another, is the most common reason for anger. The time factor is, in fact, one of the greatest restrictions imposed on man's will. The action done, the event realized, are beyond any human power. To make undone what has been done is often enough the heart's desire, never to be fulfilled. In anger more forcibly than in any reflection and analysis man is made aware of the inexorability inherent in the laws of matter and of time. But he is also made aware of the fact that he himself is part of this reality which so stubbornly refuses to be subjected. He is made aware of the fact that the laws governing reality govern his own existence too.

To repeat this once more: when passion has taken hold of the mind, such an awareness does not arise in consciousness. But the experience from which the reflecting mind can elaborate and, as it were, extract such an insight is real in the emotional situation of anger. The same is true, respectively, of all other emotions if they reach a certain intensity. If they are not so intense as to fill the whole mind, expelling all reasoning and all reflection, such an insight may develop also while emotion lasts. On the other hand, the deeper the emotion, the greater the chance that the mind, retrospectively, becomes aware of the facts revealed.

When man realizes that he is a part of reality, and at the same time that he is unique as an individual person and as a representative of rationality in the realm of being, he is enabled to develop another, very different attitude in regard to reality, the attitude namely of love. This word is so ambiguous that it is exceedingly difficult to deal with its object. First, love has been given so vague a significance by common language that its true meaning is rather obscured. People use the word indiscriminately for referring to a mere liking, say of some food, and for the highest emotion uniting friend and friend, lover and beloved, man and God. Secondly, many ways of using the word rest on a *denominatio a potiori*. This is true of Plato's Eros, as well as of *amor* in Aquinas. The *amor naturalis* is love only by analogy. Plato, however, and even more the medieval writers, had in mind the highest and purest forms of love when they gave this term so wide a signification. In modem times one kind of love, namely the love arising between the two sexes, has been considered as the only true and the primary love, of which all other forms of love are modifications or derivatives. This view is developed to an extreme in psychoanalysis.

It is true that love, in the full and strict sense, can be spoken of only in regard to persons. Love between man and woman is, therefore, true love. But from this it does not follow that this particular kind of love is the origin of all other kinds. This naturalistic misinterpretation has been criticized by Scheler and by others. True love may be said to be characterized by the following features: true love desires the highest good of the beloved; it is, therefore, by its very nature, not only desirous but is compelled to give. Its other fundamental traits are best summarized in the statement contained in the chapter *De Caritate* in the treatise *De Adhaerendo Deo.*[14] This passage reads as follows: Love draws the lover outside himself and puts him in the place of the beloved; and he who loves is more with the person loved than with self. (*Trahit enim amor amantem extra se et collocat eum in locum amati; et plus est qui amat ubi amat quam ubi animat*). These words, then, indicate the ecstatic nature of true love, its movement towards the beloved, and its tendency to unite itself with the beloved. No detailed analysis of love can be attempted here. Nor is it the intention of this article to contribute to descriptive psychology of emotional states. Their description is of interest only in so far as it makes visible somehow the "cognitive aspect."

If dread emphatically makes man aware of his nothingness, his finitude and contingency, love assures him of his being and worth. The lover loves to give, and only what has worth can make gifts. "*Bonum diffusivum sui*" not only points out a characteristic of goodness; it states also the only source from which any giving can originate. He who can give and whose gifts are appreciated, is assured of his worth, and with this, because of the convertibility of being and value, he is also assured of his true being. The nothingness which, contrary to what Heidegger pretends, is not outside of man, but inside, rooted in his very being, is overcome and, as it were, neutralized in love.

This tendency to give is not a mere "expression" of love; it is love's nature. Desiring the good of the beloved necessarily brings forth the

14 Contained among the works of St. Albert, but, in fact, as M. Grabmann has shown, by John of Kastl, a Benedictine who wrote at the end of the fourteenth or in the early fifteenth century. *Mittelalterliches Geistesleben,* Vol. I. Munich: M. Hueber, 1926, pp. 489-525.

will of having the beloved participate in every good oneself highly appreciates. The incapacity of the beloved to participate may become a serious hindrance to love. Some say that it is silly for two people "made for each other" not to marry because one, for instance, is an ardent admirer of music whereas the other remains cold to the greatest compositions. It is not so silly, after all. Love wants to give, and this means, where no tangible good is in question, to share. Love may become crippled if it is deprived of its fundamental manifestations. True, many marriages between people who are widely different and do not share all interests, likings, and "loves," are happy enough. One may, however, doubt whether these marriages realize all the happiness of which the two people are actually capable.

Much may be learned in regard to these things from the observation of children. They have nothing "real" to give; they are not able to do great things, they have not many possessions of their own, and those they have they know to have come from the very persons they love and to whom they desire to demonstrate their love. They feel a strong need of such demonstration, which is in fact more than a mere demonstration. Most of the human emotions, perhaps one may go farther and say most of the performances of the mind, reach their full completion and actuality only if they become externalized in one way or another. But if a child acquires something of his own, something not given to him, but, for instance, found, he will bring it to his mother or father and make of the thing a gift. A colored pebble it may be, or some other insignificant object. The innate wisdom of love has taught parents not to reject such a gift and not to judge it from their own viewpoint, but to enter into the spirit of the child, to admire what he admires, to praise what he gives. It is a serious and sometimes even disastrous mistake to make fun of a child's childish gifts. By appreciating them you give the child a renewed assurance of his personal worth. This is the more necessary as without such a certainty the worth of other persons becomes hidden to the child's and, later, the, adult's mind.

In this sense, then, love is the true antagonist of dread (as Kierkegaard has seen). Dread isolates, love unites. A faint reminiscence of this opposition between love and dread seems to be at work in the instinctual clinging to others so often observed in states of dread. But the clinging of dread is of a nature widely different from the nature of love's clinging. The first is exacting, and expresses a never satisfied, because essentially incapable of satisfaction, demand; the latter is essentially giving and taking at the same time, expression of the movement towards oneness, characteristic of love.

To assert that the main features of love apply also to hatred sounds paradoxical, but only as long as one does not penetrate beneath the surface of appearances. In fact, hatred constitutes as strong a bond between the hater and the hated as does love between the lover and the beloved. A life filled with hatred for a certain person may be emptied of its significance if this person disappears. The void created under such circumstances, even when the death of the hated person has been brought about by the hater himself, may become so intense that hatred originally aimed at one person may spread) as it were, to others.

Hatred is the opposite of love on the level of human relations. But dread is the opposite of both, of course of love more than of hatred, because it isolates and separates the individual from his likes. Hatred may become also a bond uniting several people against one hated person (conspiracy). Hatred is less antagonistic to dread because it eventually leads to increasing isolation. It has a corrosive power, and destroys, sometimes gradually, all loving relations, leaving the individual alone with his hatred. This may be one of the reasons why there is often disunity among conspirators. The apparent reasons seem to be others, like envy, ambition, and the like. Common hate, after all, constitutes a unity directed at an extrinsic goal, while love links one person directly to the others.

Love is said to be blind. Doting mothers are unaware of even the greatest defects in their children. A lover "idealizes" the beloved person, so much so that he appears to her eyes as the paragon of everything, however mediocre and insignificant, if not worse, he may appear to the outsider. The blindness of love is accused of bringing about many disappointments and disillusions. The gloriole of the beloved vanishes often very quickly. Marriages of love, remarked the sceptical Montaigne, more often end with disaster than do marriages of reason. In the latter case there is an objective evaluation of the other; one enters the married life with open eyes, not enraptured by passion and trusting a totally phantasmagoric image, created by oneself.

However, this generally accepted statement on the blindness of love is in need of correction. Scheler has emphatically protested against this belief, and he claims that "love makes seeing." The present writer too has pointed out that love does not always blind, and that it may even be particularly sharpsighted, in a definite sense.[15]

One thing love sees much more clearly than the objective and disinterested eye of the casual observer. Love discovers the potentialities of the beloved. Its illusion often consists in taking for actualities what is still potential. And its guilt is often that, because of this illusion, it forgets the task of striving for the highest good of the beloved, that is, for his perfection and, therefore, the actualization of his potentialities. In fact, without some attitude of love one never would discover the values of persons or of things. Love itself is no means of cognition of objects, not even of personal values, but it is, so to speak, the medium in which such a cognition becomes possible. Love makes pervious to the positive aspect of reality the mind which else may remain utterly unaware of goodness, beauty, all kinds of values. Similarly, hatred and its modifications, envy or jealousy, also make sharpsighted. Notwithstanding its will to detract, to deny values in the envied person, envy reluctantly is forced to acknowledge these values. It actually lives by this reluctant recognition.

One may, perhaps, add that the achievement of love is the correlate, on the level of philosophical anthropology, to the commandment of love in morals and faith. Only by loving himself man may become aware of the values he represents, however insignificant and humble his personality and station may appear to him. Psychology teaches us how great a handicap the loss of the awareness of self value becomes in the establishment of social relations. He who is not sure of his self value cannot truly love; he "has nothing to give" since he doubts the value of himself and love demands that he give himself. Thus, self love, in the correct sense of the term, is indeed the basis on which love of one's neighbor alone can develop. H. Bergson is right when he remarks that true hatred of mankind, true misanthropy, arises only when a man has first learned to hate himself.

While love reveals to man his own value, it also makes him aware of his obligations in regard to his fellows. The mere intellectual realization of the indebtedness to others and the fact that the actualization of human potentialities requires most of all the influence of the human and social agents is not sufficient for producing a truly effective sense

15 M. Scheler, *op. cit.*, note (12); R. Allers, *Psychologie des Geschlechtslebens*, Munich, Reinhardt, 1922, also in: *Handbuch der vergleichenden Psychologie*, ed. G. Kafka, vol. III, ibid.

of obligation. Such a sense develops only if there is a concrete awareness of the ontological equality and the moral solidarity of mankind. To accept one's place within this uniform multitude, it is necessary again to be sure of one's personal value.

Although the role of emotions has been very much misunderstood by those who emphasize the furthering of emotional reactions in education, they have seen something of truth. Without at least some emotionality, knowledge remains largely ineffective. Being sure of self value, man can also, without apprehending this as a threat for his value and existence, recognize values higher than his own. Without the capacity for love, true admiration and respect hardly develop. Both these emotional states are responses to, and at the same time conditions of, the recognition of higher values.

Related to admiration is wonder. To "explain" wonder as an effect of an alleged "instinct of curiosity" is an enterprise condemned to failure. Besides the questionableness of the notion of "instinct" there are other reasons for discarding such a simplistic interpretation.[16] Wonder results, eventually, in a movement of curiosity and an attempt to clarify the wondrous facts. But wonder is first, and curiosity second. Plato saw more clearly than these defenders of instinct when he claimed that wonder was the beginning of wisdom. In the attitude of wonder man also is made aware of his limitations, but this awareness is different from the depressive one by which man is referred back to his finitude. Wonder reveals to him the greatness of being and, to some extent, his own greatness too. It is man's prerogative that he may ask questions.

The list of examples cannot be prolonged indefinitely. Interesting and conclusive though a complete list of emotions and their analysis in regard to the thesis might be, it would mean a previous survey of all emotions and an attempt to group them according to some basic principle. This is feasible, but makes necessary a discussion too long to be attempted here. Only two further emotions, therefore, will be mentioned.

Compassion is not based, as many believe, on the realization of hardships or sufferings which may strike oneself, but on those envisioned in another. Compassion is a realization of the pain suffered by another

---

16 On instinct see: K. Goldstein, *The Organism*. New York: Amer. Book Co., 1939, and by the same: *Human Nature in the Light of Psychopathology*, William James Lectures, Cambridge, Mass: Harvard University Press, 1940. Furthermore Bierens de Haan, *Der Instinkt*, Leiden: 1940.

as this other's. It does not become fictitious for all its object being another person's suffering. Compassion also must be distinguished from the emotions aroused by a tragedy witnessed on the stage. The real suffering of a fellow being lacks the "cathartic" power Aristotle attributes to the tragedy produced on the stage. True compassion is neither to be confused with the shudder we feel when faced with misfortune, pain, suffering of all kinds, and even less with the shudder of disgust. These other emotions very often color compassion and deprive it of its pure and original nature. The frequency of their admixture, however, does not alter the essential nature of compassion. Nor must the note of condescension, of superiority, which so easily is added to compassion lead us astray. The healthy person feels, whether he wants to feel this way or not, superior to the sick and disabled person. He who is able to give alms because of his means, hardly can fail to feel superior to him who receives. It is quite significant that apparently throughout all forms of civilization the suppliant assumes a posture placing him "below" the man capable of helping. The tendency for and the longing for superiority are so strong in man that they often destroy all true compassion.

A man may help another without feeling compassion. He may do so out of a sense of duty or obligation, or because he considers such an action as according to his own dignity – noblesse oblige – or because the aspect of suffering is painful to him and he wants to be relieved himself more than to relieve the other. True compassion probably is rare. But so are all great and true emotions. The term "genius" has often been used in regard to emotional capacities. There are, according to this idea, people who are particularly gifted in the way of emotional reactions, as others are in regard to intellectual, scientific, artistic, or political achievements. In fact, the individual differences regarding emotional reagibility are hardly less, and perhaps are even more marked, than those regarding other powers of the mind. The persons capable of true compassion are exceptions.

This, however, does not diminish the importance of compassion for an understanding of the place held by emotions in human existence. The emotional dullness of the many is as little an objection against the interpretation of emotions attempted here as the incapacity for understanding higher mathematics or abstract speculation is an argument against listing such capacity among the powers of the human mind. One suspects that the emotional dullness is, with many, due less to an original incapacity than to other factors, among which the fear of further consequences and the preference for an undisturbed life play a prominent role.

Compassion unquestionably makes man aware of the general fate of mankind. While dread and some other emotions reveal to man his individual, personal finitude, compassion makes him realize the finitude of mankind in general. Being more than simple contemplation of and shuddering at another person's suffering – which attitude leaves man in isolation – it contributes to the realization of mankind's solidarity. It ensures the individual of his "belongingness." He realizes himself as a member of the great community of mankind. It is revelatory that views which deny the equality of men also incline towards a devaluation of compassion, which such ideologies consider as weakness, sentimentality, and unworthy of the "heroic mind."[17]

The second emotion, the comments on which close this brief summary, deserves particular attention. Disgust[18] is aroused whenever we see, or smell, or taste certain things, eventually also when we touch them, especially slimy, cold things. It is, however, doubtful whether all these reactions, related though they be, are of the same nature. It is possible that a distinction must be made between disgust as a true emotion and the kind of impression we call nauseating.

Nausea is, primarily, a mere vegetative reaction by which the organism responds to substances which do not agree with the stomach. Nausea is a general state in which unpleasant sensation on the part of the stomach, vomiting, or at least the tendency for it, stands in the foreground. The other bodily symptoms, such as faintness, cold perspiration, general feeling of dis ease, seem to be secondary phenomena. The close relations obtaining between the oral cavity, the sense of taste, tactual sensations, deglutition, on one hand, and the functions of the stomach – as shown by the various secretory reflexes released from the mouth – on the other hand, supply an explanation for the fact that there are also nauseating tastes, even if no experience of them

17 For a complete and penetrating analysis of compassion, see Max Scheler's work referred to in note (12).

18 There are very few studies on disgust. G. Kafka's article: "Zur Psychologie des Ekels," *Zschr. Ang. Psych.*, XXXIV (1929), 1, deserves mention, although the theory proposed therein – namely that disgust is ultimately related to and rooted in sexuality – is unacceptable. Cf. J. Hirsch, *Ekel und Abscheu*, *ibid.*, 472.

has been had before. In most case, however, the nauseating influence of tastes or smells seems to rest on association and previous experience. It has been repeatedly observed that children show little reluctance against things which an adult would qualify as nauseating.

The emotion of disgust is apparently conditioned mostly by visual and tactual impressions. If the purely sensory factors of these impressions are considered, there is little which can explain the particular effect they have on most people. Coolness and sliminess, for example, are sensations like many others, and it is not intelligible why they should acquire such a peculiar note. Nor is, say, a carrion, if considered as a mere complex of visual impressions, anything more than color, shape, and location. Still more incomprehensible is, if only the mere *sensa* are considered, the disgust many people experience when seeing blood.

The reaction of disgust seems to be primarily related to decaying organic matter or any part of an organism separated from the whole to which it belongs. An amputated limb is felt by many as a disgusting thing while it has nothing of such a quality when still in its place in the organism. Wounds are disgusting because they strongly suggest the corruptibility of organic matter; they become the more so the more the note of decay is visible (suppuration). The clean wound as resulting from the knife of the surgeon is less disgusting than a torn and irregular wound resulting from an accident. The same hair we admire on a woman may appear disgusting if we see it fallen out and separated from the head of which it is an ornament.

One can hardly doubt that disgusting objects remind man of his corruptibility. The situation depicted often by the poets and sculptors of the later Middle Ages, and shown also in several famous paintings of the early Renaissance, gives expression to this idea: a tombstone representing a corpse in decay, snakes and worms peering out of the chest covered only with remainders of flesh, and the inscription: "Thus I look, you will look the same"; the *Trionfo della morte* in the Campo Santo at Pisa, said to be a work of Traini, showing people, richly clad, on horseback, shuddering before an open grave and its content; the legend also of Buddha who escaped his guardians and, the first time he left the precincts of his castle, encountered a man sick, an old man, and a corpse, and thus was made aware, by this single experience, of the futility and uncertainty of earthly things.

With some people everything reminding them of decay or disintegration takes on the character of the disgusting: To them, a sick person, whatever his ailment, is essentially disgusting. Decaying matter and disintegrating wholes become meaningless. Chemists and physicians have often been said to lack the "natural" reaction of disgust, because they do not hesitate to handle things which to others are definitely disgusting. Partly this is, of course, the effect of habit. But partly it is also due to the fact that the disgusting things are not devoid of meaning to those students. It is not mere callousness which may make a physician speak of "a beautiful cancer." It has been said that "a chemical substance out of place is dirt, while dirt as a subject of chemical investigation is a substance." Something out of place is meaningless; whatever is meaningful, because belonging to a greater whole, loses the quality of disgustingness.

The experience of disgust thus points out, as it were, to man the value of wholeness. It does so, indeed, by contrast. But this is not an unusual fact. We appreciate innocence especially by the experience of guilt, health especially by the experience of sickness, and the possession of many things especially when and because we are threatened with losing them or actually have lost them.

One feature in the behavior of disgust deserves notice. The individual feeling disgusted draws back from the disgusting thing as if it were dangerous or, at least, threatening with contamination. Actually, the disgusting thing seldom is in any sense dangerous or harmful. On the other hand, there is a close relation between dread and disgust. Some people are thrown, by the experience of disgust, into a state of mind closely resembling dread. Disgust may become, with some, so intense that they faint or are unable to move. Heidegger might say that behind the decaying matter dwells the Nought. This is true to a certain extent, but it is hardly all.

Disgust refers to possibilities of decay and decline. It is not without deeper signification that we call "disgusting" a man's behavior which lowers him below the level of average humanity. The dissolute, the drunkard, the sloven, and so forth are "disgusting" because they place before our eyes such a possibility. Some people consider disgusting all kinds of animals. This reaction is observed also in regard to apes, those animals which appear as an infrahuman caricature of human nature. It is also noteworthy that the range of what is qualified as disgusting varies considerably with individuals and, especially, with their station in life or the demands they make on themselves and others. The attitude of moral primness which so easily degenerates into pharisaism conceives of many things as disgusting which to another mentality are not so. As it is with morals so it is with many other things. The concepts of cleanliness vary considerably, and what to one person is sufficiently clean is disgustingly dirty to another. In this attitude the positive aspect of disgust becomes apparent. The line defining what is conceived of as disgusting also defines, so to speak, the person's worth and station.

Disgust thus becomes an opposite of admiration. If the first reveals possibilities of human nature below ourselves, admiration makes us envision possibilities above ourselves. But both are possibilities of human nature in which everyone participates. The admirable achievement or the personality deserving admiration is, therefore, of a comforting nature, even if we do not think that we can attain the same height of perfection. That there are saints and heroes at all gives us more confidence in human nature, and thus implicitly in our own.

The present discussion seems to have reached the point where a preliminary summary becomes permissible. It is not claimed that the conception of emotions suggested here defines emotion in every respect. It must be admitted that emotions have other functions besides *revealing to man something of his "ontic status."* But it is claimed that this aspect of emotions is of a great importance.

The mere experiencing of emotions is not equivalent to a full knowledge of their ontological import. Such a knowledge develops only if the awareness supplied by emotional states is lifted, as it were, to the level of reflection. In regard to this, emotion is much the same as sensory awareness. The mere *sensa* have not any significance; a *sensum* as such is meaningless. It becomes significant only when synthesized with others, and also with memories and, most important, with intellectual notions. A thing merely sensed is just there. Only when it is recognized as such does it become meaningful. Recognition as such means more, in human life, than the awareness that something has been "seen before." Recognition is expressed by calling the thing sensed "a" thing of such or such a nature. Even if it is to the perceiving mind not more than "a thing," its "somethingness" is an abstract notion. Similarly, "emotional cognition" does not supply the mind with any definite knowledge unless it be combined with reflection.

The re presentation of emotional states encounters great difficulties. It is even questionable whether such a re presentation exists at all. Many have pointed out that remembering an emotional situation means living through it a second time. The "objective" data of the situation may be recalled and imagined, but the emotion is not an emotion recalled; it is a truly reproduced emotion, that is, actually present. Although the intensity of emotion may be much less in the case of representation, it is often enough sufficient to create a state of mind equalling the one which existed in the actual experience. There are also many instances of emotions of a great intensity being released by purely imaginary situations. (This phenomenon makes desirable an analysis of emotional states referring to personal, actual or fictitious, experiences and emotions referring to other persons, as for instance when witnessing a play. This problem, however, is too complicated to be approached here.)

Consideration should be given to a feature of emotional states which, as it seems, has not yet found the attention it deserves. Common language often speaks of "deep" or of "shallow" emotions. The same terms are, it is true, used also in reference to insight; one person is credited with a deeper in sight into some matter than another possesses. We speak furthermore of deep and shallow as attributes of personalities. But it seems that depth is a property primarily of emotions. We are "deeply" moved. Depth seems to have different significations when applied to knowledge and to emotions. Depth of knowledge refers to the structure of things knowable. He has a deeper knowledge who knows more about the relation of the fact considered with other facts. The more one knows about causal relations, about the significance of phenomena and their interconnections, the deeper knowledge one has. Depth when spoken of in regard to emotions, however, does not refer to the "objective" world, but to the person affected. Depth is not of layers of reality – or ideality, as the case may be, briefly of the "non ego" – but of the subject himself.[19] It would seem that the expression "depth" is, indeed, more appropriate when applied to emotions than to any other experience. "Deeper" insight or knowledge, in the usual sense, is, in fact, "broader," encompasses a greater number of relations between different terms. It is questionable whether the use of "layer" and, corre-

19 It is hardly necessary to point out that the depth referred to here has nothing to do with the depth of which "depth psychology" boasts. The depth of which this psychology, e.g., psychoanalysis, speaks is of the same nature as is depth of knowledge. The "layers" psychoanalysis considers as building up human personality are conceived in terms of science and not of experience.

spondingly, of "depth" in regard to the objects of science is legitimate.[20] Ontologically speaking, what is below the surface is the realm of substantial being which unquestionably is beyond the grasp of science. There is only one point in the whole field of possible experience where the knowing mind grasps, although hardly in an adequate manner, substance itself, and this is in self experience. Self experience does not mean, in this sense, introspection, not even an introspective analysis directed at "functions" or "acts." Although this kind of self experience is exceedingly valuable, much more so than certain psychologists, blinded by their ideal of a so-called scientific psychology, are willing to admit, it is not the immediate awareness of the being self. The being self remains, as it were, still behind, or beneath, the acts apprehended by even the most careful introspection. It is in "deep" emotional states that consciousness grasps something of the self's very being.[21]

In reviewing some of the current theories on emotions, those pretending to give some "explanation" in terms of biology may be discarded. There is, in this regard, little progress since Callicles proposed

20 Thus far one may agree with the claim made by the "Circle of Vienna" in a programmatic pamphlet stating the general intentions of the group: "Science," they wrote, "knows of no depth; it keeps strictly to the surface of phenomena." Science, in the strict sense in which this term is used, may indeed not be able to penetrate below the "surface." But this statement has a philosophical significance only if it is previously assumed that knowledge exists only by and within science. Such a statement, however, is itself no longer of science but of philosophy. A thinker who denies to science, justly, the capacity of seeing below the surface and at the same time asserts that science is the only legitimate form of knowledge, commits a serious logical fallacy, and speaks of things of which he, by his own principles, cannot know anything.

21 This explains why so many people have a definite aversion against all kinds of deeper emotion and take pains to escape any situation which might result in their being truly and deeply moved. They are deadly afraid of meeting themselves. Kierkegaard has some very pertinent remarks on this matter too. The means by which any such experience is avoided are manifold. To describe them is the task of psychology, or anthropology. The less anyone is sure of being a true person or of possessing true worth, the more will he endeavor to escape the "descent into the hell of self knowledge," to use an expression by which Kant named what he deemed to be the necessary condition for any ascent to a higher knowledge or form of existence.

the theory of pleasure as a repair or restoration after "depletion."[22] Nor need those conceptions be considered which make emotions indicative of the helpful or harmful. These too are old. Originally the reference was to a higher state of perfection (as in Spinoza: Pleasure is the passage of man from a lesser to a greater perfection). An age which has learned to regard the purely vital functions as the only relevant ones and is dominated by materialism is bound, of course, to distort the original meaning.

The so called definitions devised by H. Spencer for pleasure and pain and, in wider application, for emotions in general, are no definitions but simple restatements of what is observable to everyone.[23] The criticism to which these alleged definitions were subjected by several authors[24] proved no reason against repeating the same platitudes. Thus E. L. Thorndike speaks, instead of pleasure and pain, of satisfying and annoying stimuli. Satisfying means "those states of affairs which, in the case of human beings, are welcomed, cherished, preferred to exist rather than not to exist."[25]

Not much more useful are the theories which connect emotions with "frustration." If by this is meant that emotions arise when an appetitive movement does not immediately find an outlet, there is some truth in the conception, although it does not cover all cases. Especially, such a theory falls to explain the joy of possession. Incidentally, this conception too has its predecessors, for instance in the idea of Herbart that emotions result from the mutual inhibition of "ideas."

The psychological study of emotions has suffered by the general prejudice that "feelings," pleasure and pain, must be considered as the simpler and more elementary phenomena and that the "higher" emotions accordingly must be analyzed into such feelings plus some either factors. This conception starts with the unproven assumption that

22 *Gorgias*, 494b; see also *Timaeus*, 64a 65b; Aristotle, *Ethica Nicomachica*, VII, 14, 1154a25 ff. Only such theories are considered which have some bearing on the particular problem under discussion.

23 H. Spencer, *Principles of Psychology*, 3d ed., New York, 1896, Vol. I, p. 250.

24 E.g., H. R. Marshall, *Pain, Pleasure, and Aesthetics*, New York, 1894.

25 E. L. Thorndike, "A Pragmatic Substitute for Free Will." *Essays in Honor of W. James*, New York, 1908, p. 588. The tautological nature of this "definition" has been pointed out, for instance, by H. Cason, "The Pleasure Pain Theory of Learning," *Psychological Review*, XXXIX (1932), 440.

"simple feelings" are the same under all circumstances, that is, that there is only one kind of pleasantness or unpleasantness. Recent researches, however, have shown that even "simple" pleasure may be qualitatively different. Pleasure of satisfaction is of another nature than pleasure of function (as found in play activity) or pleasure of creation.[26]

However, the authors dealing with emotions, notwithstanding the differences of interpretation, are agreed on one point: emotions are subjective states, that is, they have no direct reference to the objective world. They are indicative, to consciousness, not of situations without, but of situations within. They are considered as "states" of the subject, or the manifestations of such states to consciousness. They are not *gegenständlich*, but *zuständlich*.[27]

The nature of emotions as modes of the subject is referred to in various manners according to the general conception of the authors. Introspection, says R. S. Woodworth, "renders attractive" although not evident the conclusion that feelings are reactive attitudes of the organism.[28] F. Krueger states that emotions are distinct from all other modes of experience but are in connection with them; they are "complex qualities of the actually existing totality of experience.[29] A. Willwoll sides with Krueger, as do many other authors, for instance Stieler.[30] A particular feature emphasized by E. Raitz de Prentz is the passivity of emotions. They are subjective and arise in consequence of impressions or situations without any activity on the part of the subject, as pure responses.[31] One is reminded of the concept of *passiones animae*, which term, as one knows, refers in a narrower sense to emotional

26 To have consistently disregarded these facts is one of the serious mistakes psychoanalysts make. They consider pleasure of satisfaction, as corresponding to the attainment of an instinctual aim, the only form of pleasure. Cf. the present writer's comments on this point, *The Successful Error*, New York, 1940, Sheed and Ward, p. 137.

27 This feature may be absent in simple feelings, especially of the sensory kind. But emotions are modes of the person, notwithstanding their reference to objective facts or situations.

28 R. S. Woodworth, *Experimental Psychology*, New York, 1939, H. Holt.

29 F. Krueger, *Des Wesen der Gefühle*, Leipzig, 1837, p. 118.

30 A. Willwoll, *Seele und Geist*, Freiburg i. B., Herder, 1938, p. 119; G. Stieler, "Die Emotionen," *Arch. f. d. gesamte Psychologie*, 1925, L, 343.

31 E. Raitz de Frents, "Bedeutung, Ursprung und Sein der Gefühle," *Scholastik*, 1927, II, 402.

states, although it has a general signification too. It is true that even in a purely receptive attitude the mind is more spontaneously active than in emotions. Perception entails activity at least in so far as there is a turning towards the object, a paying attention to it, and so forth.

There is, however, another property of emotions which, perhaps, is more characteristic and allows us to penetrate more into the nature of these mental states than mere passivity. Psychologists apparently have hardly noticed this property of emotion, but it has been pointed out by E. Husserl. While all other mental phenomena, especially those of cognition, present to the reflecting mind various aspects or sides, this peculiarity is found missing in emotions. Husserl, to describe the changing aspects of other mental phenomena, uses the term *abschatten*, that is, being differently shaded, or appearing in different shades. Nothing of the sort is discoverable in emotions. "If I look at an emotion, I have something absolute, it has no sides which might present themselves as such at one time and otherwise at another time. I may think truly or falsely about an emotion, but what stands before the look is absolutely there in its qualities, intensity, and so on."[32]

Nor can it be denied that in this "absolute" the mind is aware of a modification, not so much of itself, but of that of which the mind itself is part and manifestation. Husserl emphasized even more forcibly than Descartes had done the certainty of the *ego cogitans*. In this sense he stands within the great tradition stemming from St. Augustine's *scio me scire* and leading, without any interruption, down to Descartes and to all the philosophers influenced by him. It was more than courtesy shown to the French institutions that had invited him which made Husserl call his lectures at Paris *Méditations Cartésiennes*.[33]

The expression "modifications of the subject" or of the ego, if one prefers, is still in need of clarification. 'What modifies the ego, so that it becomes cognizant of its being modified? The note of passivity inherent to emotional states indicates that these modifications somehow come from "without." This "without" must not be taken in a spatial sense. It designates the whole realm of the non ego, including therefore not only things and persons, but truths and values too. On the other hand, emotional states are in peculiar manner personal and "subjective." The latter term has been given, in modern philosophy, a

32 E. Husserl, *Ideen zu einer reinen Phaenomenologie und phaenomenologischen Philosophie*, Halle, a. S., M. Niemeyer, 1913, p. 81.

33 E. Husserl, *Méditations Cartésiennes*, Paris, A. Colin, 1931.

depreciating note, quite undeservedly. The subjective experience can be considered of lesser value or importance only if it has been previously ascertained that "public knowledge," capable of verification by everyone wielding the appropriate methods, is superior to any other knowledge under all conditions. This contention is much less "self evident" than the empiricist believes. The whole question of the relative worth and importance of the "subjective" and the "objective" has, therefore, to be examined anew. This examination should be the first task of empiricism. With this school rests the burden of proof, as is always the case whenever philosophy pretends to correct and supersede the evidence of common sense. It is not enough simply to declare that any statement not subject to "verification," fashioned according to the pattern of science, is *ipso facto* "meaningless." As long as this claim has not been founded on some evident principle it is "meaningless" itself, because it cannot be proven by any kind of experiment. This must be kept in mind if one desires to defend the right of any psychology not of the "scientific" type. Discussions as carried on here are considered inacceptable by those who are addicted to the idolatry of science and disregard all other forms of experience.

Since emotions are modifications of the experience the ego has of itself, they are, at least in this fundamental aspect, beyond the grasp of "scientific" psychology. Accordingly, the perusal of the textbooks and of periodicals filled with the studies of experimentalists proves fruitless if the reader is looking for some information on the nature of emotional states. However "objective" and "scientific," the psychologists cannot help being aware of the existence and the role of emotions. Some restrict their statements to the outward manifestation of emotions, bodily changes and behavior; others consider the total situation in which the organism develops an emotional reaction. Some allow even certain data of introspection to creep in. The result of their observations and ideas reads about this way: Emotions ensue whenever the organism is placed in a situation which has some bearing on its welfare. Emotions of lesser intensity prove helpful; if too intense they may become a hindrance to adequate reaction. Of middle intensity they are reinforcing agents for appetitive or conative behavior. They are indicative of "interests," of the useful and harmful, or, with man, of any sort of value.

Is there any relation between the generally accepted interpretation of emotions and the conceptions tentatively submitted on the foregoing pages? The answer depends on the idea one forms of the situations to which the organism, or rather the person – since we do not know anything of emotional states in animals, of which we can observe only behavior resembling our own when experiencing emotion – responds by an emotion. According to the thesis defended here, these situations must be of such a nature as to provoke a realization of the "ontic status" of man in general and of the individual person in particular.

In this regard it is noteworthy that emotions develop with age, and that there is a definite parallelism of cognitive and emotional capacities. This is to say that emotions become more differentiated the greater the capacity for distinction between situations becomes. In the newborn infant and up to an age of about three months one observes only a general pattern of excitement.[34] At the age of three months the reaction patterns of distress, excitement, and delight are clearly distinguishable. Distress is differentiated, around the age of six edge of other bodies. Somesthesia, after all, is one of the achievements of sensory organization, and it may well be that here too a sensible species (*species sensibilis*) and the whole process of sensory awareness enter into play. We have, in fact, an image of our own body, although it is usually not clearly developed. But it underlies all our knowledge regarding the postures of the body and the localization of stimuli affecting the body in some spot, and may become disturbed by pathological processes.[35]

Awareness of the body, however, is not awareness of self. When we know ourselves thinking, we have no direct knowledge of any bodily functions being involved. It does not matter whether or not the brain is active in thinking, either as the "organ of thought" or as supplying the sensorial basis for abstract thought. The main point is that man is conscious of his thinking without knowing anything of his brain. Also, we know our bodies as "ours," as "belonging" to ourselves. The self may be confused, in common language, with the body. But phrases

34 G. M. Stratton, "Excitement as Undifferentiated Emotion," *Symposium On Feeling and Emotions*, ed. C. Murchison, Worcester, Mass., 1928, Clark University Press.

35 Many years ago the present writer described such disturbances of "autotopognosis." The image of one's own body, as a frame of reference for our consciousness of posture, etc., has been called, by others, the "body schema." R. Allers, "Uber Störungen der Orientierung am eigenen Körper," *Zentralblatt f. Nervenheilkunde*, 1909.

like "I have burned my hand," reveal the awareness of truth's existing also in the average, non reflecting, unsophisticated mind.

The facts have been somewhat obscured by the Cartesian proposition, especially by the ergo. This word implies that man knows himself to be because he thinks. The state of things is apparently better described by saying: *cogito cogitationes meas* – I think my thoughts. In fact, every one of our thoughts – or, generally speaking, of our mental states – is directly and unmistakably characterized as "mine." There is no need for reflection on this fact; it is primarily and absolutely evident. There is no way of even "methodologically" doubting the fact that every mental state observed directly is my own. The Augustinian formula "I know that it is I who knows" (*scio me scire*) renders the facts better than the Cartesian proposition.[36]

This knowledge or awareness of one's self, however, is of a peculiar kind. It is, immediately, only awareness of being (or of existence, to use this term of certain recent philosophies). Existence as such is in no way determined; existence is simple "thereness" or *Dasein*, as Heidegger says. This philosopher, indeed, makes the attempt to characterize existence by certain properties, or features, or whatever term seems appropriate Heidegger is perfectly conscious that all these terms connote meanings he wants to be excluded. He, therefore, coins for these determinations of existence the term "existentials." From this, incidentally, it becomes clear that one misinterprets Heidegger's notion of existence if one sees in it the same as the *esse* or *existere* in Scholasticism and other traditional philosophies. (The relations between *esse* and *Dasein* and the shape the whole question of the real distinction between essence and existence takes on in Heidegger's philosophy are very much in need of clarification.)

'What Heidegger overlooks is that besides these so called "existentials" there are other determinations – or at least one such determination – which are fundamentally important. Perhaps he does not overlook this fact, but deprives it, because of his general outlook, of its significance. The fact referred to is that man is conscious of worth. The term conscious must not be unduly stressed. It is not the same con-

36 In recent times R. Hönigswald has emphasized the basic importance of the fact "I know that I know" and of the indefinite prolongation of which this statement is capable. Of course, there is no actual infinite regress, because the "I know" is on every step the same. Cf. *Prinzipien der Denkpsychologie*, 2d ed., Leipzig, Teubner, 1928.

sciousness by which we know, for instance, a tangible fact or a thinkable truth. One might speak of a "co consciousness," comparable to the knowledge of the ego, which in Kant's words must accompany all our mental acts. This ego is not only there, not only being, but also being gifted with a definite worth.

Worth or value implies a relation. This is not to be understood in the trite, and false, sense that value refers to a relation obtaining between a subject and an object, as if things had value only "for me." The relation alluded to here is one obtaining between values. No value is apprehended in perfect isolation. All evaluation entails an outlook on the total order of values.

It has been too little recognized that our judgments of values and of their height rest on considerations different from most others which allow any kind of scaling or rating. Magnitudes are judged by means of some unit in comparison with which these magnitudes are greater or smaller. The term "unit" does not mean that in all estimations we refer to a known and measurable unit; but the procedure of estimation is of the same kind as if we applied a yardstick. In evaluation, however, we proceed quite differently. Magnitude in the common sense starts from a zero point; the first step beyond this point defines the unit. Evaluation knows of no such zero. There is no zero of moral goodness or aesthetic beauty. Nor can one say, in a meaningful manner, that one moral or aesthetic value is so many times greater than some other value. The "measures" of aesthetic values by accidental factors, such as the number of people who like the object under consideration, or the price paid for a painting, the copies sold of a book, and so forth, are no true "measures" of aesthetic values.

What do we mean when we say, e.g., that a painting by Tintoretto rates higher than one by Carracci, or that Shakespeare's plays are "better" than Massinger's? Many will answer that such an utterance indicates simply the greater pleasure we derive from one of the two things submitted to comparison. Even superficial observation is enough to disprove this statement, notwithstanding its incessant repetition by authors of renown. It is a compliment to the taste and understanding of the public if a work of great art is liked by many, but to be liked by many is not necessarily a criterion of great art. Were this the case, greatness of art would become utterly relative, so that what was great art yesterday is no longer so today, but may rise to the former height tomorrow The nonsense of such an opinion is still more evident if one turns to moral values.

The judgment on values rests on a very curious process which may be called the "appreciation starting from the maximum." Man carries with himself, somehow, an "idea" of an absolute value, representing the maximum of each class of values, absolute beauty, absolute goodness. By declaring a painting very beautiful, we do not state that it is distant by so many steps from the zero of beauty, but that it approaches more than any other work the "ideal beauty," although we have never experienced this ideal, nor ever will, at least not in this sublunar world. The same is true of goodness.

Every value of which we become aware is placed, automatically as it were, somewhere on a scale, the upper end of which serves as starting point. A valuable thing is not simply valuable, but it is always so much valuable, that is, it is always put in relation to the maximum of value.[37]

Although the estimation starting from the maximum is, perhaps, characteristic of evaluation only, the fact that a given object denotes, in itself, its place in the order to which it belongs, is not exceptional. It is rather the general aspect of cognition. A sense impression need not be of the utmost, hardly tolerable intensity to be apprehended as very strong. One may suppose that a person who never saw any other shade of red besides a pale pink would be able to conceive of a greater redness although he might be quite incapable of imagining such a shade. There are analogies to the *via eminentiae* on all levels of being and of experience.[38]

37 It seems possible to construct, by making use of these and other facts of evaluation, an "axiological" demonstration of the existence of God. Such an attempt has been made by M. Scheler, *Der Formalismus in der Ethik und die materiale Wertethik*, Halle a. S., Niemeyer, 1916. The reasonings of this philosopher, however, are marred by his misunderstanding of the ideas of *summum bonum* and *ens realissimum*. He in fact contends that axiological reflection leads to the notion of *summum bonum*, while metaphysical speculation ends with the concept of *ens realissimum*, but that there is no convincing evidence, in reason, to be found for the identity of the two. The lack of clarity in these points explains somewhat that Scheler, later, arrived at the impossible conception of a God in development; *Die Stellung des Menschen im Kosmos*, Darmstadt, 1929, Reichel.

38 The facts alluded to here were, as far as the present writer can ascertain, first emphasized by J. Pikler in a series of *Schriften zur Anpassungstheorie*

Self-evaluation implies, therefore, an apprehension, however imperfect it be, of the place the individual holds, as embodying a definite value, in the order of values, the special order of "personal" and the order of values in general. But value does not exist by itself; it is the value of some being. By evaluating something we assign to it a place not only in the order of values but also in the order of being. It is even so that our judgment on the ontological position of some being rests more on evaluation or the value we apprehend as belonging to the thing than on a comprehensive analysis of the properties of the thing. We are guided in such a factual analysis by the value which we apprehended.

These evaluations follow their own laws which defy, in a way, "rational," that is, any, demonstration comparable to the methods of science. There are evident principles which cannot be reduced to more fundamental ones. Thus, the obvious superiority of persons above things is an evident principle. It can be correlated, of course, to ontological or metaphysical principles. But if we say that, e.g., the human person possesses the greatest dignity among all material things, because of his rational nature, we are led to ask what are the foundations of the greater dignity of the rational nature. And proceeding further, we arrive at statements which assert the greater worth of a simple, a spiritual, an immortal substance, or the greater worth of the cognition of universals, or the greater worth of self determination. Ultimately we have to recur to last and evident principles of evaluation.[39]

However, the fact that evaluation is back of the most fundamental insights does not amount to asserting that value or goodness is prior to being or truth. Although such an opinion may be maintained, and

des Empfindungsvorganges, especially one discussing Weber's law, Leipzig, 1919 1929, Barth. See also Ch. Hartshorne, *Philosophy and Psychology of Sensation*, Chicago, 1934, University of Chicago Press; J. P. Ledvina, *A Philosophy and Psychology of Sensation, with Special Reference to Vision*, Washington, D. C., 1941, Catholic University of America Press. Apparently without being influenced by the few psychologists who held such views, D. W. Pratt has developed a similar interpretation of sensations, especially in the field of audition. See his *Aesthetic Analysis*, New York, 1936, Cromwell.

39 Those last principles cannot be discussed here. Although one may not agree with his statement in all points, the remarks of M. Scheler on this point, in his great work on ethics, deserve fullest attention.

has been maintained,[40] it cannot be demonstrated by a mere reference to acts of the human mind or, if one prefers, of the human person. Evaluation and its proper object, value, may be prior only with regard to ourselves.

Thus, it seems that evaluation is at the bottom of all our attitudes in regard to reality, including our own self.[41] Evaluation, however, must be considered as a true cognitive operation; it cannot be located in the appetitive powers. One may, if one likes, call it "preconscient," although it is probably more correct to speak of a pre reflective or unreflected cognition. There is no doubt that unreflected cognition, not only of values, holds an important place in human life. A great part of our performances, our orientation to our surroundings, and similar traits of conduct are either originally unreflected, or have become so by secondary automatization. The impressions received by the senses are immediately utilized for regulating behavior, without being made the object of reflection.

One ought to distinguish between "preconscious" and unreflected processes of the mind. Mental events on which reason does not throw its light are not yet, for this reason, "unconscious" or "preconscious." The failure to discriminate between the various levels of mental performances – especially the sensory and the rational level – has induced many to extend unduly the field of the "unconscious." Much has been

40 The ideas submitted in this article have a certain resemblance, as this writer discovered while casting his essay into its final form, to the views of H. Guthrie, *Introduction au problème de l'histoire de la philosophie*, Paris, 1937, Alcan. The resemblance is, this writer feels, more apparent than real. The particular ontological conceptions of Dr. Guthrie cannot be considered here. A careful analysis would be needed to arrive at a sufficient clarity in regard to Dr. Guthrie's notion of a priority of value as set over against what he calls the mathematico-logical approach in philosophy. In the present context, we have to deal exclusively with the cognitive aspect of emotions and with ontology only in so far as certain references to metaphysics may help to a better understanding of the reasons why emotional states play such a prominent role in a full realization of man's "ontic" situation.

41 This seems, on further reflection, to be necessarily so. Evaluation being the achievement of the *vis cogitativa*, which not only co operates in forming the final shape of sensory awareness and the phantasm but as *ratio particularis* is an essential factor in all particular actions, is the very pivot of attitude and behavior. Its cognitive achievements, therefore, cannot but be at the bottom of all attitudes in regard to reality.

called by this name which, in truth, is not unconscious but subrational, not "outside" of consciousness, but simply not fully realized, since such realization entails reflection and, therefore, an operation on the part of the rational faculties.

The fact of unreflected cognition or awareness implies a further peculiarity which also may give rise to an objection against the views submitted. Emotional responses are not only "irrational" in the sense that they are independent of and previous to any intellectual control. They are "irrational" also in the sense of being quite often unreasonable, unfounded, and meeting disapproval from others as well as from oneself.

Emotions are not judged by their own standards. An action is judged according to the principles regulating action in general; it is considered right or wrong. A statement is true or false, according to principles of the concrete or the abstract order. An emotion, however, is justified or not. It is neither true nor false, neither right nor wrong in itself. It is "in correspondence" with the objective situation, or not. The kind of situation is not a content averred by the emotion itself, but is ascertained by an analysis generally subsequent, achieved by the cognitive powers. It is wrong to feel glad because of the misfortune of another; but gladness felt as such is not wrong, nor is it right. It is wrong only under the given circumstances. It is justified if one feels grief because of the loss of a dear person; it is not justified to he sad because of the loss of a "beloved "object. Grief itself, however, is neither justified nor unjustified. Thus, emotions do not know of any intrinsic regulative principle. They are given their place in an order which is not itself emotional or directly related to emotion. The order according to which emotions are said to be justified or not is the order of either the moral or the aesthetic values.[42]

42 The facts referred to above constitute, as may be remarked parenthetically, an objection which cannot be met by any theory making values dependent, in their cognition and their existence, on emotions. If it were the emotion itself which constitutes value, the fact of an "unjustified" emotion could not be observed at all.

It may be that the joy a person eventually feels because of the fall of his enemy differs in kind from the joy the same person feels when meeting his beloved. The existence of such qualitative differences may be assumed in consideration of the strict correlation of the objective and subjective sides in mental phenomena. But this is not the question. The question is rather whether the individual, while experiencing such a joy, is aware of any dif-

There can be no doubt that emotions often occur without an objective situation supplying a sufficient reason for this type of emotional response, or for any type. This fact seems to make questionable the view proposed here, namely, that man, in emotion, becomes aware of his "ontic status." If emotions are so frequently out of place and not of the right kind, they cannot be considered as a reliable source of any kind of awareness. Furthermore, emotions are called "merely subjective" for several reasons, among which one has to be referred to in this context. To the same objective situation different men respond very differently. Emotion as a state by which man becomes cognizant of his "ontic status," would reveal different aspects to each individual.

This objection, however, may be met by two considerations.

First, one must be careful not to confuse" objectivity" of a cognitive process with "reliability." A cognitive performance may be beset by many dangers of error, and yet reveal, under certain conditions, the true state of things and thus be "objective." The fact that mistakes or errors occur is, in itself, no decisive argument against any method or procedure.

---

ference. That this is not the case can be surmised from many observations and also from the lack of a correspondent vocabulary.

The judgment others or, eventually, the subject himself, may pass on such an "unjustified" emotion is not founded on another emotion. If we feel unpleasant because we reacted in an unjustified manner, we feel this way because of the judgment we formed on our behavior. But the judgment is not based on a second emotion.

These considerations have, incidentally, a bearing on the much discussed question of the role of emotions and their education. To develop emotionality, or the capacity of emotional reactions, to pay attention to the child's emotions, is right only if, at the same time, care is taken that the emotions arise on occasions which justify such a reaction. There is no sense in developing, e.g., a capacity of enthusiasm if the mind is not directed toward the things which deserve enthusiasm.

Aesthetic reactions without a cultivated taste and an understanding of true art are of no value.

Since man easily reacts emotionally to situations which, by their nature, do not warrant such a reaction, control is as important as development. There are many instances in which to remain unmoved is wrong. But there are probably not fewer in which to react emotionally is unjustified, or which demand another kind of emotional response than the uneducated mind is likely to give.

Secondly, the unreliability of emotions, taken in their cognitive aspect, may not exist at all. There need not be a strict correlation between certain objectively defined situations and equally well defined emotions. For man to become aware, in the medium of an emotional state, of his "ontic status" the only condition is that there be emotions. The "ontic status" is, in fact, prior to and independent of any particular situation. This status, accordingly, is immutably the same whatever the situation. Even an unjustified emotion may reveal this status. The revealing power, e.g., of shame, is the same whether one is ashamed because he committed a sin, or because he was guilty of a breach of conventional rules. Whether or not the particular emotional response is justified does not abolish the fact that an emotion of this or that nature has been experienced. Whether we fear an imagined or a real danger, fear is in both cases the same experience. Or as a famous psychiatrist once put it: "If you dream of a tiger, the tiger is fictitious, but the fear is real." We may love a person "unworthy our love." But what love can reveal to us in regard to the" ontic status" of man may become apparent whatever the nature of the beloved and however unfounded our attitude may be.

There are further emotional attitudes which, by their very nature, are always and essentially unjustified, like hatred. Hatred, in the true meaning of the term, is directed against persons. We "hate" other objects only in a metaphorical sense, either by personifying them (as we may "hate" a horse which is the cause of an accident to a beloved person), or by using the word "hatred" instead of the more correct "abhor." The sentiment of hatred may also spread from a hated person to other things related to him, just as love makes valuable and loveable things which we associate with the beloved, like a token of remembrance. Although totally unjustified, these emotions may reveal something of the "ontic status" of man.

It is quite correct to speak of emotions as "subjective" states. They have no direct reference to the objects which are known by the cognitive powers. One really ought to devise a particular term for designating the "object" of which emotional states mediate the cognition.[43]

43 A. v. Meinong tried to overcome a similar terminological difficulty. He uses the name "object" for the intentional correlate of perception, and the name "objective" for the correlate of judgments (*das Objectiv*). To orective states corresponds the "desiderative," and to emotions, as has been remarked before, the "dignitative." Since the theory of "emotional presenta-

The subjectivity of emotions, thus, cannot be made into an argument against the cognitive function envisioned here. What is cognized is not that by which the particular emotion is actually released. Justified or not, the emotion retains its character and with it its ontic reference.

Another objection, however, apparently carries more weight. There are emotions which may be called "spurious" and may be said to lack the feature of a "genuine" mental state. The notion of genuine and non genuine mental states has been proposed by W. Haas and A. Pfaender. A genuine state is one in which the person lives, as it were, in his totality, while a non-genuine mental state allows for the various "layers" of consciousness to remain unintegrated. A man who is assiduously devoting all his attention to his work, but in whose mind there is some constant worry, for example, about his child sick at home, is in a non genuine state. This term does not connote any evaluation; it is purely descriptive. Nor does this term imply any difference in "intensity"; a man may be more attentive in a non genuine manner than another is in a genuine manner.

There is however a certain type of non genuine emotions in which much of their true nature is lost. What is alluded to may be best exemplified by the habit or attitude of "sentimentality." A sentimental person not only reacts emotionally in an unjustified manner – that is, out of proportion with the actual event releasing the emotion – but his emotions are felt by the observer to be shallow, and somehow distorted, as if they were turned from their original and appropriate direction by a secret agent within this person's mind. The impression of shallowness may, curiously enough, persist notwithstanding a great display of emotional manifestations. This is true also of certain abnormal personalities, usually qualified as "hysterical."

---

tion" of values seems inacceptable to the present writer, he cannot adopt Meinong's terms. But the attempt of the Austrian philosopher deserves to be repeated. A good deal of misunderstanding probably could be avoided, if "object" were not used indiscriminately for sensed things and intellectually apprehended relation, between terms (*Sachverhalte*), and in many other ways too. The "existential" of Heidegger cannot be used either, because of the particular connotations this term has in this philosopher's system. The knowledge mediated by emotion does not, as interpreted here, refer to any "features" or "characteristics" of existence or the existent being in itself, but to the place this being holds within the order of being in general, especially viewed as the order of *bona*. The present writer admits that his endeavors to devise a suitable name have failed.

The emotions of the sentimental person are non genuine because this type is so self centered and so much addicted to a continuous contemplation of himself – frequently in the manner of self pity – that he never is capable of a truly integrated state of consciousness. The emotional state never really gets hold of such a person. His way of experiencing emotions is paralleled by the way certain people seemingly enjoy art, music, or poetry, whereas in truth the only thing they enjoy is their capacity of enjoying. They are, to put it rather crudely, continuously admiring themselves for their understanding of art, etc. It is as if they were continuously saying to themselves: "How wonderfully do I appreciate this." And thus, they are focused mainly on themselves and not at all on the object. This object is to them a mere opportunity for displaying, chiefly before the audience of their own consciousness, their capacity for appreciation. The sentimental person behaves much in the same manner. One only has to listen to his repeated assurances that his is an exceedingly emotional and sensitive nature to become aware of the strong element of egocentrism. The emotional reactions of such sentimental people are often inadequate, out of proportion. They will weep bitter tears, for instance, because of the suffering of animals, object emphatically and unreasonably against any kind of experiment performed on "the poor rabbit," and be utterly unmoved by the fact that there are children starving, people living in crowded slums.

Everyone presumably knows such types. They impress even the casual observer as artificial, untrue, as play actors. They themselves, however, believe in the depth and the genuineness of their emotions. If, however, these emotions are not really what they are believed to be, can they reveal to such individuals anything about their ontic position? A negative answer imposes itself. But, then, how can anyone trust his emotions? If the sentimental person deceives himself, everyone may be in the same situation. He may know as little as the sentimental individual about the reality of his emotions. Anyone relying on whatever knowledge he may gather by means of his emotional experiences may be seriously misled and arrive at notions lacking all objective validity. Consequently, all conclusions drawn from emotional experience are not to be relied upon, and must be discarded. To this reasoning one may counter that the same distinction pointed out before, applies here too, namely the one between objectivity and reliability.

Secondly, it has to be admitted that not every experience qualified as deep and genuine emotion by the subject can be credited with these properties. It may be true that there are no sure criteria by which a subject would be enabled to ascertain the genuineness of his emotions, although even this allows for certain restrictions. But there is the fact that non-genuine and shallow emotions are recognized as such by the observer. Of course not by any observer, and perhaps by none in some cases. The mere fact, however, that such a "diagnosis" is possible at all ought to make us doubt the assertion that no reliable criteria may be found.

One of these criteria consists in the effect emotion has on the total life and the personality of him who experiences the emotion. By way of illustration one may refer to the well known error of naturalistic alienists in considering as pathological all tears, for instance, because of the suffering of animals, object emphatically and unreasonably against any kind of experiment performed on "the poor rabbit," and be utterly unmoved by the fact that there are children starving, people living in crowded slums.

Everyone presumably knows such types. They impress even the casual observer as artificial, untrue, as play actors. They themselves, however, believe in the depth and the genuineness of their emotions. If, however, these emotions are not really what they are believed to be, can they reveal to such individuals anything about their ontic position? A negative answer imposes itself. But, then, how can anyone trust his emotions? If the sentimental person deceives himself, everyone may be in the same situation. He may know as little as the sentimental individual about the reality of his emotions. Anyone relying on whatever knowledge he may gather by means of his emotional experiences may be seriously misled and arrive at notions lacking all objective validity. Consequently, all conclusions drawn from emotional experience are not to be relied upon, and must be discarded. To this reasoning one may counter that the same distinction pointed out before, applies here too, namely the one between objectivity and reliability.

Secondly, it has to be admitted that not every experience qualified as deep and genuine emotion by the subject can be credited with these properties. It may be true that there are no sure criteria by which a subject would be enabled to ascertain the genuineness of his emotions, although even this allows for certain restrictions. But there is the fact that non genuine and shallow emotions are recognized as such by the observer. Of course not by any observer, and perhaps by none in some cases. The mere fact, however, that such a "diagnosis" is possible at all ought to make us doubt the assertion that no reliable criteria may be found.

One of these criteria consists in the effect emotion has on the total life and the personality of him who experiences the emotion. By way of illustration one may refer to the well known error of naturalistic alienists in considering as pathological all kinds of visions or ecstatic phenomenon, simply because states, apparently of the same nature, occur in mentally diseased people. However, there is an enormous difference. The ecstatic state of supernatural origin – or even a natural ecstasis as occurs sometimes with artists – results in a heightening of life, in a further step onwards and upwards in unfolding of personality, an enrichment of the mind. The pathological state, on the other hand, is a symptom of progressing disintegration of personality.[44]

Similarly, true and genuine emotions, even those of a depressive nature, have, or at least may have, a positive influence on personality. Sorrow and grief often have deepened a man's understanding of himself and of human nature. Non genuine emotions have no such influence. The sentimental personality does not become richer, deeper, more perfect, by indulging in those non genuine emotions. Rather, the longer this habit persists, the more superficial such a person becomes. Also, he gradually loses the capacity for true appreciation of values. Everything appears to him as equally important, because he reacts on the most insignificant events with what he considers a deep emotion. Thus, he is unable to react with a greater intensity when a serious reason arises, because he has, so to speak, spent his emotional energy

---

44 One of the most striking examples of this incapacity for appreciating things not strictly of the psychiatrist's special field may he found in Dr. G. Zilboorg's new book, *A History of Medical Psychology*, New York, 1942, Norton. This author does not hesitate to qualify Socrates, of all men, a schizophrenic because he "heard voices," the voice of his *daimonion*. Up to now we were used to seeing the naturalistic psychiatrist talk of the neurotic and psychotic states of saints; now the philosophers are getting their diagnosis too. However, it must be emphasized that not all psychiatrists, even if they are far from say belief in things supernatural, commit such silly and superficial mistakes. The famous French psychiatrist P. Janet, for instance, acknowledged that no hysterical personality can develop the character nor be capable of the achievements of which the life of St. Teresa of Jesus gives testimony.

on so many petty occasions. He deplored the loss of a pet so much that his reaction cannot be any stronger when his mother dies. Such a degeneration of the sense of values cannot but become conducive towards a gradual impoverishment of personality.

True, fully developed and genuine emotions are probably as rare as all other perfect things are. Not every person is capable of experiencing emotion so that his experience would become a true revelation of the "ontic status." This, however, does not deny the capacity of such a knowledge to those who, because of nature or because of other reasons, are incapable of deep and genuine emotions. Not the fact that an emotion does not reach a perfect stage, but mistaking the imperfect state for the real thing, is the great obstacle.[45] Man somehow is aware of the fundamental role played by emotions in his life, and he is often somehow although hardly admitting this to himself ashamed of lacking higher emotionality. He may turn this defect into a virtue and become a stoic. Or he may close his eyes to the fact and convince himself that his very imperfect emotional experiences are all one may expect. If, however, he realizes where he stands, he may attain the same knowledge as anyone capable of the most intense and deep emotional responses.

Reference may be made, in this context, to a point touched upon before. Every kind of experience which exists in different degrees enables the mind to conceive of degrees not actually experienced. (The psychological as well as the ontological aspect of the *via eminentiae* deserves a closer study than can be given it here. But the fact is easily ascertained, even though its interpretation, on the psychological and the ontological level, may present some difficulties.) This "extrapolation" beyond the degree actually experienced enables man to grasp, if in a less impressive, but still in an adequate manner, the true nature of the emotion he experiences. The only condition – but it is one hard to fulfill – is that a man be perfectly honest in regard to himself and that he be willing to subject even his emotions to an examination so as to find out whether they are genuine and justified, or lacking genuineness and related to objects not justifying the kind of response. The great obstacle is, of course, man's vanity. This is the more the case, since

45 It is hardly necessary to point out that "perfection" as used here refers exclusively to the state of full development. A thing is perfect if it is all it can be by its nature. No moral connotation, of course, is intended.

emotion, by being characterized as subjective and personal, seems to "belong" more to the person himself than ideas, images, concepts, and suchlike phenomena, which are related to the objective world. Man dislikes acknowledging that he has been deceived by appearances, or mistaken in his judgment; but he dislikes more acknowledging that his "feelings" are wrong.

It seems well to emphasize once more that the emotional state does not in itself supply a true knowledge of the "ontic status." Emotion is only the medium by which (the id quo) such a cognition becomes possible. The cognition results from a subsequent reflection on the emotional state and its "objective reference." There are analogies to this in the field of sensory knowledge. A mere awareness of *sensa,* or of the senses being somehow affected, does not amount to cognition.

Although, e.g., the threat of infinite power, the impending or, at least, possible annihilation of the contingent and finite being is "given in" the emotion of dread, this implication becomes a content of consciousness only by way of reflection. Nothing, therefore, could be more mistaken than to displace or even only to devaluate the importance of reason for man, governing his life and perfecting his personality. To the contrary, reason remains the only guiding light which enables us to see things as they are, their universal nature, and to envision purposes and goals for our will to achieve.

One further question has to be considered briefly. It may seem, at first sight, as if by speaking of a "cognitive aspect" of emotional states a new form of cognition were suggested for which no place can be found in the system of traditional psychology. It seems as if a cognitive faculty were postulated of which the generally accepted theory is ignorant. This impression, however, rests on a misunderstanding. Not only does the view submitted in this article not introduce any new faculty of the cognitive order, but this view can be maintained in a consistent manner only if the notions on the faculties of human nature are maintained just as they are taught by traditional psychology.

Emotions (or the *passiones animae*) arise – according to traditional interpretation – as correlates to the movement of the sensory appetites. These appetites are aroused by the awareness of goods or evils, envisioned in the particular object or situation actually confronting the individual. This awareness is the achievement of the cogitative power (*vis cogitativa*). This internal sense, then, is the faculty which mediates the cognition implied in emotion. It has been shown elsewhere (see note 1) that evaluation is a performance of the *vis cogitativa*. Any apprehension under the aspect of goodness rests on the activity of this faculty. This has been overlooked and certain authors have been forced by this neglect into rather amazing construction, as, e.g., crediting the appetitive faculties with a cognitive capacity.

A. certain doubt may prevail regarding the origin of the awareness of self value. It is hardly possible that a sense, even one of the internal senses, should be able to make the person himself an object of cognition. However, this problem differs in no way from the other of the awareness of individual existence.[46]

Before summarizing the views suggested, tentatively, it seems advisable here to point out that the role of emotions already considered is not the only one these mental states play in the total economy of man's life and his relations to the non ego. Emotions fulfill several other tasks.

A cognition of values by means of emotional states, crediting them with "intentionality" is a fiction, forced on certain philosophers and psychologists by their incapacity to account otherwise for the apprehension of values. Here the notion of the *vis cogitativa* fills an important place which is left empty by the modern psychological conceptions. The fact, however, that emotions as such are not id quo values are known does not prevent them from wielding a great influence on our attitude in regard to values. There is a mutual influence (flowing to and fro, so to speak) of emotions and the correlated movements of

46 Any more detailed discussion of the origin of our knowledge about ourselves is excluded here. Such a discussion would mean a thorough analysis of the many factors which have been credited with the capacity for furnishing the mind with such a knowledge. *Somesthesia* chiefly has been made responsible, although there are several reasons which discountenance such a theory. For the ends envisioned in this article it is sufficient to point out that a knowledge of self value is in no way more mysterious – which does not mean that there is no mystery involved – than a knowledge of self existence. Perhaps it is an ultimate fact, not susceptible to any further analysis or elucidation, that man simply knows himself as existing and as having a certain worth. The problem, then, becomes not how man knows of his existence and worth simpliciter, but how he arrives at an opinion on his existence as related to other existing beings, and on his worth as compared with the order of values, especially personal values. On this latter problem the discussions of the foregoing pages, this writer ventures to hope, did throw some light.

the sensitive appetites on one hand, and the performance of the *vis cogitativa* on the other. The value aspect of things apprehended by this power releases an orective movement, and the corresponding emotion, in turn, makes the cognitive faculty more pervious to the value object. Although values may be recognized without any emotional response ensuing, there is no doubt that these values are apprehended with greater clarity if such a response takes place. Of this fact, an explanation may be given in the terms of the views suggested here. However, a discussion of this point is better reserved for another place.

Secondly, emotions act on the appetites as reinforcing factors. It is, perhaps, not possible to state in a general manner anything about the priority of emotion and movements of the appetites as conscious phenomena. Apparently, there are instances in which the mind is conscious first of an emotion and then of some longing, which then is said to be conditioned by the emotional state; and there are instances in which the sequence seems to be reversed, the longing or desiring[47] arising first, and the emotion following.

In the latter case, emotion is definitely experienced as strengthening the orective movement. This seems even to be the main function of emotion. It acts, if such a comparison seems permissible, much as a reinforcing valve in a radio set.

The weak currents arriving at the receiving part of the set (the antenna) are reinforced so that they can cause audible vibrations in the effector part, i.e., the loudspeaker. Emotions as such are hardly ever the motive agents which determine action or behavior (with the exception, of course, of purely expressive forms of behavior). The causes of action are the values as apprehended in the objective world or the non ego. But these values, as apprehended, usually possess too little dynamic force to release any kind of energic action. Their efficacy has to be rendered greater by the intervention, or intercalation, of emotions. This is especially true of values which must be apprehended as something more than a reaction to mere pleasantness.

Some authors, among whom M. Scheler and N. Hartmann deserve mention, hold that the higher a value is the less capable it becomes of determining behavior. This is true in way of description, but does

47 It would be well if the relation of "desire" in the usual sense of the word, and of *desiderium*, as listed by Aquinas among the *passiones animae*, could be clarified. But this matter too must be discarded because of the lengthy analysis it demands.

not, as these philosophers assume, state anything on the nature of the higher values or, for that matter, of any value. In fact, rare though such instances are, we know of people to whom a value such as theoretical truth appeals at least as strongly as sensuous values appeal to the majority of average personalities. Still rare, but more numerous than the cases referred to before, are those who react with a noticeable intensity on high moral values, people to whom the suffering of their fellow creatures "means more" than the greatest achievement of art or the most intense sensuous pleasure, or even the gratification of vanity.

Since exceptions do not confirm, but rather invalidate any rule, we may safely assert that there is no rule stating the inefficacy of higher values. It is not the higher values which are ineffective, it is the human person who is irresponsive. These, obviously, are totally different assertions: the efficacy of the higher values is denied, not absolutely, but only in certain cases (not simpliciter, but only *secundum quid*).

Some people who have developed a particularly thorough understanding of values may act according to this understanding alone, without emotion intervening. But these are exceptional cases. The average person reacts on values only if a corresponding emotion of sufficient strength is aroused. In so far it is indeed desirable that emotions be considered in education, but it is a mistake to make the development of emotional life as such a goal of educational measures.

The least important aspect of emotions is doubtless the one which has been considered fundamental by many more or less naturalistically minded philosophers, the aspect namely which connects emotion with stimuli or situations furthering or endangering life. This may be true in some instances, it may be true particularly of brutes, but it is assuredly not generally true of man. Most of the emotional states of man have no direct reference to the preservation or furthering of life. Such a relation has to be constructed, and usually is constructed on the basis of evolutionistic notions. Whether or not such an explanation is sound need not be investigated here. From the viewpoint of descriptive psychology, at least, there is hardly any indication of such a connection.

To summarize briefly the main ideas submitted in the foregoing pages: It is submitted that emotions make apparent to the mind the "ontic status" of man, that is, the place he holds within the order of being. This knowledge, as it is mediated by emotion, is unreflected and reaches clarity and definiteness only by reflection on the whole of the emotional situation when, subsequently, the intellect is focused on this situation. The cognitive aspect of emotion does not belong to the emotion as such but to the cogitative power, the apprehensions of which release the emotional state. The proper object of this apprehension is the value side of being. Values are not apprehended simply as this or that value, but always and necessarily as values of this or that height. A good of a lower order is not taken for the highest possible good, even if no higher good has been as yet experienced. To this connotation of the place held by a value datum there are analogies also in other fields of experience.

Emotion, however, does not simply reveal the value aspect of some object or situation. This is done effectively by the *vis cogitativa*, whether or not an emotional response ensues. Emotions have been characterized as "merely subjective." This is not true, inasmuch as they have some kind of "objective reference." It is true, however, inasmuch as emotional states reveal the particular relation of the subject to the order of values and thus the subject's own value.

Man is capable of attaining a view of his "ontic status" also by mere reasoning without emotion necessarily intervening. The impressiveness of a more immediate or experimental awareness is, of course, much greater. In this lies one part of the importance a well developed emotional life has for the unfolding of personality. Mere emotion, a mere indulging in emotional upheavals, without the clarifying activity of reflection being added, is more harmful than good. However important emotion may be, it is still the light of reason which proves the only reliable guide.

Emotions, as revelations of the "ontic status," point mainly at the finiteness of human nature. If what they reveal is correctly understood, man becomes more conscious of his position as a creature, a contingent and finite being. At the same time, he is relieved from the depressing idea the knowledge of finiteness, contingency, and utter dependence may condition. He then realizes that nowhere has his position been defined better than in the words of the Eighth Psalm: "What is man?" Man is nothing; he is not worthy that God be mindful of him. Yet he has been made a little less than the angels. His position is so high in the order of created being that he nearly reaches the level of the angelic nature.

While the depressive and, generally speaking, negative emotions reveal to man his nothingness, his true "not being" – as compared with

Being Itself – other emotions assure him of his worth. Dread, threatening with annihilation and revealing its intrinsic possibility, forcibly points out to man his finiteness, limitation, his being nothing, although he be somehow. But love, and all other emotions which reveal to man his capacity of worth, his chance of growth, and the indestructibility of his worth, notwithstanding the acknowledgment of values greater than those he may call his, these emotions mean not only enhancement of vitality, not only joy and pleasure, but also the glad recognition of the order of values within which man holds, paradoxically, such a prominent place.

Rudolf Otto, in his book on *The Holy* speaks of the various aspects of Divine nature: God as the *mysterium tremendum*, the *mysterium fascinosum*, and so forth. Rational speculation may indeed lead us to similar conceptions. But we tremble not simply because we know that there is a reason for trembling, and we do not love simply because we know that there is a reason to love. Our faith may be intellectually perfect, and yet be "cold." Rational conviction may be sufficient for will to determine itself towards an act of faith and the obedience to divine law. Reason may also convince us of the finiteness of our nature and of the existence of God. Reason, thus, may become conducive also to conversion. And faith need not be less strong, conviction not less deeply rooted, willingness to comply with the commandments not less effective, for all lack of emotional response. Emotion is not a *conditio sine qua non* for religious life. If it were, no constancy and continuity of this life could be guaranteed, since emotion depends on so many factors beyond all control by conscious will.

On the other hand, a well developed emotional life may contribute much to the deepening of religious attitudes. It is not in vain that, for instance, the gift of tears is listed among the particular graces accorded by God to some elect persons. Nor is it without a profound significance that the saints were, generally speaking, as great in regard to their emotional responses as in regard to other achievements. The poetic joyfulness of St. Francis of Assisi, the quaint humor of St. Philip Neri, the ardent love for poor and suffering people so universally characteristic of saintly personalities, like many other features known in hagiography, need only be mentioned to make evident the close relation between a perfect life and a capacity for sound emotional response.

Emotional response, however, is sound when it is "justified," that is, proportionate to the objective situation to which it responds. A mere cultivation of emotionality, as an end in itself, will cause more harm than good in the advance toward the perfect life. Emotion too, whatever its importance, its spontaneity, its impressiveness, must be subjected to the control of the rational faculties. It is not emotion itself which decides on its rightness or wrongness. Such judgment is passed by reason only. Here as everywhere it is right reason to which the ultimate judgment belongs, and it is good will to which belongs execution.

THE LIMITATIONS OF MEDICAL PSYCHOLOGY

Medical psychology has gained a great influence in many fields. Terms taken from the various schools are used by all kinds of writers. Psychologists and. sociologists, writers of fiction and of educational treatises, and authors dealing with politics or with history speak of repressions or inferiority complexes, of compensation, of sublimation, of the collective unconscious or the disastrous consequences of frustration. Many of these expressions have become part of everyday language. The infiltration by terms originating in medical psychology has proceeded at an astonishing rate. It took much longer for terms of science to penetrate our language.

It is interesting to inquire into the causes of this success.

But it is perhaps even more important to raise the *quaestio iuris*, and to ask whether or not such a reception of medical psychology is justified.

Every branch of knowledge has definite boundaries, outside of which special notions and categories either lose their literal sense or produce distortion and falsification in the field where they are illegitimately employed. The boundaries may not be perfectly visible and, especially in a discipline still in its youth, may often be badly defined. In such cases there is need of clarification. Unfortunately, on the part of some scholars there is a tendency to oppose any attempt at clarification. Animated by a spirit of imperialism, they endeavor to extend the realm of their special discipline as far as possible. They contend that principles found effective in their own field not only can but must be applied in other fields – eventually in all other fields. Scientists have often been obliged to condemn philosophers for their presumption in passing judgment on every other kind of knowledge. The criticisms were not unmerited. Philosophers have often been guilty of such imperialism. Not only the schools of Hegel and of Schelling, but some also among the Neo-Scholastics have ventured to declare "impossible" observations and theories which physicists have described or proposed. Philosophy thus lost credit and has not yet regained the esteem of its adversaries. Scientists, of course, have committed exactly the same fault. Relying on analogies which were often very superficial, they have claimed for the principles of science universal application.

The claim of the scientists has had a greater success than the claim of the philosophers. Science, at least, could point to tremendous achievements which have changed the face of the earth and the forms of human life; so that "science" and "scientific" became the catchwords of the nineteenth century. It even became a generally accepted idea that science alone supplied reliable facts, and that no branch of knowledge was worthy of consideration except in so far as it could boast of scientific methods. Hardly anyone inquired into the justice of the claim; and the success of science paved the way for a kind of new idolatry.

The human mind was one of the first fields which the imperialism of science set out to occupy. The fathers of modern psychology, G. T. Fechner and W. Wundt, cherished the hope of founding a "scientific psychology," a psychology fashioned according to the pattern of physics. Hence the former's attempt to establish a "psychophysical formula" which, so he expected, would place psychology on the same level as science, since measurement and quantification were to be introduced into psychology. Fechnerian psychophysics proved to be an illusion. Today there is scarcely a psychologist who believes that mental states can be directly measured as we measure quantities in physics.

The failure of psychophysics did not discourage the excursions of science into the still unoccupied country of psychology.

The studies carried on in laboratories of experimental psychology, although valuable, proved wholly unsatisfactory to those who expected psychology to answer questions arising in other fields. Historians and psychiatrists, students of art and literature as well as sociologists turned away from "official" psychology and began to psychologize independently of the *ex officio* psychologists. The effect was confusion. The resulting psychologies were not "scientific." They were, in fact, largely speculative. They filled the gaps of psychological knowledge with sometimes surprisingly fantastic theories. However, interest in things psychological grew, notwithstanding the confusion. A fervent admirer of Freud could prophesy that future historians would speak of our times as the "age of Freud" as one hears of the age of Galileo or of Newton. The opinion is surely exaggerated. But there is a grain of truth in the statement. Our age is, one is tempted to say, obsessed by psychology.

The reason for this remarkable phenomenon is, perhaps, not too difficult to discover. Recent times have lost the true and comprehensive conception of man's nature. The co existence of conflicting interpretations is a sufficient proof. These interpretations range from a pure materialism which considers man as a mere agglomeration of infra-atomic particles, through a mitigated naturalism which looks at man as one animal among others, to highly imaginative conceptions inspired by Indian philosophy, or other exotic ideas. In another dimension, they range from absolute individualism to a theory making the individual a mere element of a greater whole, the State, or the nation, or the race; from the picture of man as a "bundle of instincts" to a view which makes him the absolute master of his fate. And so forth.

Philosophy had lost credit with the multitudes. Only in diluted form and slowly did philosophical ideas penetrate the general mentality. Religion had dwindled to a pale deism, or had been replaced by an avowed or unavowed atheism. Science alone ruled supreme. Where could mankind find an image of itself? Science did not at once satisfy this desire; but it promised to do so. Meanwhile, burning questions which trouble and worry man's mind could not wait indefinitely for an answer. The uncertainty which was felt, however dimly, to exist everywhere, the economic and social tensions, the political threats, the uncomfortable situation preceding the first world war, created an ever increasing need for a better understanding of reality, and this meant first of all a better understanding of man himself.

At just the right time, medical psychology made its appearance. This, of course, was no mere chance. The birth of such a new discipline was characteristic of the general mentality and cultural situation at the end of the nineteenth century. It will be forever to the credit of the men who inaugurated medical psychology, in the modern sense, that they felt the necessity of developing a new conception, comprising man's physical nature, his personal characteristics, and his destiny in one view. The founders of psychoanalysis obeyed the urge of general cultural forces. This does not lessen the merit of such pioneers of the new movement as the two Viennese physicians, Breuer and Freud.

Psychoanalysis, as Freud later called his particular development of the ideas he had shared with Breuer (and in part learned from him), is but one form of medical psychology. It was the first to develop. It will not remain the only or even the most important school. Whatever Freud's disciples may want to believe, the laws of history hold for psychoanalysis. There is no final achievement in empirical knowledge, even though the psychoanalysts may feel that they are in possession of the ultimate secrets of human nature.

In this belief they show themselves true heirs of nineteenth-century scientific optimism. The question here is, however, not of the truth or value of psychoanalysis. On this matter the present writer has spoken elsewhere.[1] The psychoanalytic doctrine is referred to here only as an instance of a widespread tendency to transfer uncritically the notions and categories of medical psychology to all kinds of other fields.

This tendency is, of course, not characteristic of medical psychology alone. Psychology too has achieved a dominating position in fields where it used to be considered a merely subservient discipline. Psychology, normal or medical, today not only supplies to education means and ways, but also prescribes aims. The demands that "frustration" be avoided and that "self expression" be cultivated imply a peculiar definition of mental health and a peculiar conception of human nature in general. Yet it ought to be evident that aims or purposes can never be proposed by any purely scientific discipline. Empirical research cannot determine what ought to be.

Medicine, curative and preventive, has for its goal to preserve the health of the community. But this goal will be recognized only so long as the generally accepted ethics approves of it. We see, for instance, that in Germany the life and health of those only who "deserve" to live are to be cared for by the physician and the hygienist. Individuals who are of no value to the German people are allowed to die prematurely; or they may even be killed if they prove to be a useless burden to the community. The idea is not new in Germany. It had been proposed long before the Hitler regime came to power. Two eminent scholars, a psychiatrist and a jurist, discussed and suggested the "annihilation of worthless lives"[2] – worthless, of course, for the community – and made it clear that they considered such a measure as morally permitted or even good. Thus, the "aim" of medicine becomes different if the general "morality" takes a different turn.

Similarly it is imaginable that another age might form quite another opinion of the "danger of frustration" and consider "self expression" less

1 *The Successful Error*, New York, 1940.

2 A. Binding und A. Hoche, *Die Vernichtung lebensunwertes Lebens*, Leipzig, 1929, A. Thieme.

desirable than conformity with the generally recognized moral principles.

Categories of science, whether physics or psychology, retain their meaning and value only within the field for which they are destined and where they are, so to speak, at home. The medical psychologists, however, pretend that their methods and notions permit a better understanding of art and poetry than do the notions used by the students of these problems. There is here a grave misunderstanding. The most that psychology may eventually contribute is an understanding of why an artist painted such and such a picture at this or that period of his life, why a certain event acquired a particular significance for this individual poet, and so forth. The viewpoint is merely "physiognomical," that is, it considers the work exclusively as "expression," but not in its proper being. A work of art is something, has significance and value, even if we do not know anything of the artist's personality, let alone his "instincts." Our ignorance of such things does not, for example, diminish our admiration for Egyptian statues.

The psychologist may study the mental process of evaluation just as he studies the process of perception. But he is unable to tell us anything about the thing perceived, that is its objective nature, and equally unable to make any statement on values, whether of a work of art or of a moral action.

Notions like beauty (in aesthetics) or virtue and sin (in morals) are unattainable by the methods and categories of psychology. General psychology has become less guilty of such unjustified extensions of its field. Medical psychology has committed this error quite frequently.

The fundamental mistake made by most schools of medical psychology consists in confusing the "explanation" of the occurrence of a mental fact with a statement of the nature of the fact. Even if a psychological theory should explain why a person conceives a particular idea at a certain moment of his life, it would still leave utterly unexplained the nature of this idea. One can make it clear why an artist painted, or a poet wrote, or a scientist questioned, as they did, by referring to their past experiences, attitudes, complexes or what not; but this does not contribute anything to our understanding of the painting, the poem, the theory.

The general viewpoint of current medical psychology can be characterized as one of extreme subjectivism. Objective data, ideas, values are of no interest to this psychology. Psychoanalysis goes farthest in this. While individual psychology at least acknowledges the existence of objective laws of social life, rooted in man's nature as a social, being, Freudianism looks at all objectivity as a mere outcome of subjective forces which, ultimately, tend to one end only, the satisfaction of instinctive needs. The thoughtless adoption of such notions and theories would be a real danger for moral philosophy for education, for all endeavors which have to take account of objective facts and laws. The subjectivism of medical psychology makes their followers blind to objective values. At the best they become utilitarians, at the worst they become individualistic hedonists.

If the intrusion of medical psychology in other fields has wrought no greater havoc than it has, it is because of the inconsistency which enables so many people to harbor contradictory ideas. They go on upholding traditional standards of ethics and, at the same time, feel satisfied that they are "keeping abreast of the developments of science" by speaking and thinking in terms which are quite incompatible with the rest of their convictions.

Medical psychology has strengthened the tendency towards narrowing as far as possible the range of responsibility. Misdemeanors of all kinds, antisocial attitudes, criminality and immorality of the worst sort are comprised under the heading of neurosis, psychopathic states and similar names, all of which refer to pathological factors. A man does not misbehave or commit a crime because it is his will to do so. He cannot be made responsible. He is the unwilling victim of his inferiority complexes, of his instincts which have unfortunately been "frustrated" and which now take revenge, as it were, on the powers which, years ago, inflicted frustration.

It is clear that along with the notion of sin, the notion of virtue loses all meaning. Virtue and sin, good deeds and bad ones, can be spoken of only if there is free will and responsibility. Moral philosophy has, of course, never overlooked the fact that free will is restricted by many factors, as the past history of a person and the influences which formed his character. No doubt, many cases of criminality are due to mismanaged education, to unfavorable impressions, to a secret desire for revenge. No doubt also that the idea of inferiority may condition many forms of antisocial behavior. It is right to inquire, in each individual case, whether or not such factors are at work. But there is an enormous difference between this acknowledgment and the generalization that every case of antisocial or immoral behavior has to be traced back to such impersonal forces and that, accordingly, no one can be made responsible for his actions, be they good or bad.

Education, social sciences, law, and the other disciplines which have too often made their own the ideas of medical psychology have neglected to inquire into their reliability. They have fallen prey to the fascination of systems which boasted of being "scientific." General psychology has done likewise. The idea of basing whole systems, of psychology, theoretical and applied, on the notion of the reflex may serve as illustration. The reflex still is referred to by psychologists as a firm foundation for their theories, while this very notion has become more than questionable to the neurologist and neurophysiologist. Thus Sir Charles Sherrington has warned the psychologists and physiologists that not a single fact ascertained by the study of the nervous system warrants a physiological interpretation or "explanation" of mind.[3] The eminent physiologist arrives at the conclusion that mind is a primary factor in reality, and one that is not to be reduced to matter. It will take some time for the psychologists to become conscious that in their reflexological theories, or their stimulus-response bond conceptions, they have built on sand.

No psychology, whether medical or not, can give a satisfactory account of the contents and characteristics of mental states. Psychoanalysis, in spite of all its efforts, cannot deny that there are qualitative differences in mental phenomena which remain unexplained. Even if psychoanalysis were right in asserting that all human interests, evaluations, strivings, and so on, are transformations of instinctive longings, the question ultimately would still remain unanswerable: Whence stem the manifold varieties of interests, strivings, preferences?

Psychoanalysis and, in a lesser degree, most of the other schools of medical psychology are guilty of the fallacy of "psychologism." One would think that the devastating criticism of this set of ideas, by E. Husserl in his *Studies in Logic*, had uprooted the psychologistic fallacy from most minds. Husserl's work was published first in 1900.[4] He showed that psychology is utterly incapable of furnishing the basis of logic. And. the same is true, respectively, of factual sciences and of ideal knowledge. Mathematics does not deal with the mental processes by

3 Sir Charles Sherrington, *Man on His Nature*, New York, 1940.

4 E. Husserl, *Logische Untersuchungen*, 3d. ed. Halle 1913. Niemeyer. For an excellent summary see: E. P. Welch, *The Philosophy of Edmund Husserl*, New York, 1941, Columbia Univ. Press.

which the human mind figures out a sum or a difference. Mathematics deals with the laws of magnitudes, or other "ideal" objects. Logic does not discuss the ways by which the reasoning mind arrives at valid conclusions, but the relations obtaining between any objects in general, existing or non existing, real or ideal.

Medical psychology is essentially psychologistic. Many of the students of this discipline, in fact, claim to "explain" the nature of the objects and the relations obtaining between them. They ignore the obvious fact that these objects have to be, if the mind is to become aware of them, liking them, aiming at them, reasoning about them.

Medical psychology becomes guilty of "imperialism" once it attempts to impose its categories and ideas on other disciplines where they have no application. The preposterous claim to "explain," for instance, the logical fact of negation by the activity of some instinct is an illustration of such an unwarranted predatory excursion. Negation is either a fact, namely the awareness of something not being or not being here and now, or a category of logic. It is something the mind may think of, but not a thing the mind can create.

It must be realized that medical psychology, such as we now know it, is a child of a definite mentality which is already on the brink of the grave. It is, in a way, amusing to note that the psychoanalysts who describe the psychology of the past as the product of certain social and cultural conditions do not stop to consider the conditions which fostered the development of their own theory. Psychoanalysis belongs to an age of materialism and relativism which, we may hope, is coming to an end.

Medical psychology has contributed its part, and not a small one, to the devaluation of reason. Reason is considered as a mere epiphenomenon. Reason does not determine human action, but rather hidden instinctive forces or the inferiority complex, which from some "secret place of the heart" manages to poison the mind. In this, medical psychology, notwithstanding its positive achievements, has joined with the forces which are undermining the edifice of Western culture.

No student of abnormal minds will deny (and the present writer is far from doing so) that medical psychology has taught us many things regarding the pathology of mind and the abnormalities of behavior. Nor will it be denied that the curative methods prove useful and helpful in many cases. But it must be emphatically denied that medical psychology has supplied us with any new or tenable conception of human nature.

The facts ascertained by the medical psychologist – in so far as they are facts – find their place in a "philosophical anthropology." But they are not the whole of it. Moreover, one has to be careful regarding these so called facts. Many of them are findings stated in the language of preconceived ideas.

Thus, "resistance," so often mentioned by psychoanalysts arid others who have adopted the psychoanalytic jargon, is not a fact. The fact is that a person, during analysis, refuses to go on with the free associations or declares that there is a blank in his mind. To call this by the name of "resistance" is permissible only if the fundamental conceptions of Freudianism are previously accepted.

Nor can medical psychology ever replace ethics. Rather, medical psychology, as it exists today, is the offspring of a definite ethical theory, however much the father of psychoanalysis may have been unconscious of this dependence. Similarly, the individual psychology of Adler and G. C. Jung's modification of phychoanalysis presuppose a definite idea of ethics.

The subjectivism of medical psychology makes it impossible for those who adhere strictly to the current systems to recognize either objective truth or objective value. Truths of science exist independently of the workings of the mind, whether these be conceived as rational or as irrational (as Freud conceived them). What is good and what is evil do not depend on psychological principles. Goodness and badness are "discovered," much as facts about material things are discovered.

The continuing infiltration of medical psychology into so many fields deserves careful attention. Little harm will be done if one is conscious of the limitations of medical psychology. Great harm may result if these limitations are overlooked. Science, even if more reliable than medical psychology generally is, ought not to supersede common sense altogether. Nor ought it to replace the principles of general and moral philosophy. If the scientist adheres to a wrong philosophy, it does not matter much, since his scientific statements are independent of his philosophy. But a psychologist holding a wrong philosophy is a menace. He deals with human life directly. He claims that education and the moulding of the future generations must be fashioned according to his dictates. Medical psychology, mostly based on an inacceptable philosophy, is a real danger.

This danger is imminent. Educational psychology is full of notions derived from medical psychology. Social workers are taught the principles of psychoanalysis and told to apply them in their case work. Medical students are inculcated with psychoanalytic ideas. Medical psychology is no doubt necessary. But it should be founded on a sound philosophical basis. The misinterpretations of human nature, of man's place in the world, of the origin of truth and goodness, all these "dialectical heresies" (as St. Anselm would have called them) must be combated as best one may. Attack is never successful unless the strength of the enemy is fully known, and unless the enemy is attacked with weapons equal to his own. Not by referring to tradition, not by emphasizing the incompatibility of certain statements with principles of morals, philosophy, or religion, can the position of the materialistic, hedonistic, subjectivistic schools of medical psychology be overthrown. This can be done only by setting over against their untenable, although suggestive, assertions the unimpassioned study of facts. It is high time that medical psychology be studied – and practised by men not fettered by the prejudices of the nineteenth century and not blinded by idolatry in the face of pseudo scientific theory.

INTUITION AND ABSTRACTION

The following remarks have been suggested to me by the study of Dr. Sebastian Day's, OFM, work *Intuitive Cognition, A Key to the Significance of the Later Scholastics* (Franciscan Inst. Publ., Phil. Ser., No. 4, 1947). The author refers repeatedly to some articles of mine, critically but generously. He does me the honor to consider my ideas as representative of Neo-Thomism. I do not hold a brief either for St. Thomas or his disciples, and my reply is, therefore, not in the name of this school, but exclusively in my own.

However, I do not think that a purely polemic answer is very helpful; the idea to refute, if I am able to do so, point by point the statements of the author does not appeal to me. That I disagree with him on many and very fundamental points, is natural; were it not so, he would not have singled out my studies as a point of departure for his criticism. Simply to restate my opinions would be repetitious and not advance the discussion. It seems to me that it would be better to raise some questions, to refer to some facts, and to draw certain conclusions independently of the reasonings so ably worked out by Dr. Day.

There are chiefly two questions concerning which I wish to submit some considerations. (1) What does psychology or our understanding of intellectual operations profit, when we admit that the intellect is capable of intuiting particulars? (2) Are there any facts available which render this proposition untenable and force us either to return to the Thomistic position, that is to crediting the intellect with abstractive knowledge only, or to devise a third interpretation, better able to *salvare apparentia* and, at the same time, to avoid the admittedly existing difficulties of the Thomistic conception?

The discussion of these two questions will allow for incidental comments on one or the other of Dr. Day's statements which I believe to be erroneous.[1]

Before proceeding however with this discussion, I should like to comment briefly on a point of a more general nature.

1 I sincerely hope that Dr. Day will accept my remarks, even where they flatly contradict his position, in the same spirit in which he rightly supposed that I would read his criticisms.

As quoted above, Dr. Day's work stresses the "significance of later Scholastics," He also mentions that I have, when analyzing the Thomistic theory of intellectual knowledge of particulars, not made any reference to the views of these later Schoolmen, especially to that of Ockham. He is of course right; but I dealt there only with such conceptions with which St. Thomas himself is concerned, and views which appeared after his time seemed not to be pertinent. Dr. Day contrasts the philosophies of Duns Scotus and of Ockham with that of St. Thomas. This is obviously a legitimate procedure since philosophies may be envisioned in themselves and insofar as they are outside of historical time. Usually, account is taken of an eventual dependence of a philosopher on the knowledge of his age only insofar as factual knowledge influences his particular views. Thus, the defects of Aristotelian Scholastic physics are understood as resulting from the state of physical knowledge as it existed then. The historians of ideas, at least many of them, have abandoned the attitude of contempt which the more "progressive" minds of the seventeenth to the nineteenth century used to adopt; they have come to realize that the greatness of a philosophical conception is not de pendent on the extent of factual knowledge. They also are aware of the precariousness of a position which would consider as final the state of knowledge as it exists momentarily.[2] But when setting over against one philosophy of a later time to one preceding it, one has to take account of the changes the general mentality of the age had undergone.

Until the time of Aquinas, and at his time, the notion prevailed that the universal or general is endowed with a higher dignity than the particular. This had been, on the whole, the attitude of all ancient philosophers. It is evidenced in Plato's opposition of "opinion" and "truth" or "knowledge," It is back of the endeavors to attain clarity concerning the "existence" of the universals, that is, the conflict between "realism" and "nominalism," It has not even disappeared today; the preference given to "scientific" knowledge in contrast to all other forms; the idea that there is no real knowledge but that attained by scientific procedures, is more than reminiscent of this preference of the universal over the particular. *Scientia est de universalibus.* The goal of scientific endeavor is

2 It is amusing to read utterances of like intent in works written long ago. E.g., Gulielmus Parisiensis, speaking of one of his predecessors says, more or less: poor man, of course he was wrong, since he had not yet knowledge of the existence of the *empyreuma.*

the discovery of the universally valid law. And the desire of science to reach laws of an ever greater generality may be traced back to the same basic attitude which animated ancient and medieval speculation.

There is, however, one great difference between the "modern" and the old spirit. The former, though aiming at the discovery of universal laws, starts from the concrete particular and returns there for verification of its general propositions, whereas prior ages, all Aristotelian empiricism notwithstanding, were somewhat contemptuous of the particular fact.

The late thirteenth and the fourteenth centuries saw a great change developing. The emphasis shifted from the universal to the particular. The way problems were envisioned became different.[3] It is, therefore, not quite just to criticize an author of an older age for not having considered a viewpoint which, according to the general intellectual attitude of his time, he could not envision. Nor is it quite just to credit an author of a later time with a discovery he could not have made – if one may indulge in such a phantasy – had he lived a century earlier. To be Ockham, one needs not only Ockham's mind, one must also live at Ockham's time.

It is an interesting question to ask what factors have brought about the shift of emphasis from the universal to the particular, a process which prepared the way for the rising of science and the de cay of philosophical speculation; the latter, because the influence of Ockham notwithstanding, philosophy did not go along with the development of the general spirit. This is, however, a topic not to be discussed here.[4]

There is another general problem concerning which a few words should be said before entering into the special inquiry, if for no other reason than to introduce the argument to be presented here.

Dr. Day seems, if I am right, to conceive of a philosophical system as a context of propositions which follow strictly from some few axioms, as a system of mathematics can be thus developed.[5] It is, how-

---

3 The remarks made above may sound rather dogmatic. I realize that they are in need of ample confirmation by historical facts. I cannot, of course, attempt any further discussion of these matters.

4 Much valuable information on this point may be found in H. Heimsoeth, *Die sechs grossen Themen der abendländischen Metphysik*, 2d. ed. Berlin, 1934.

5 Cf. the work of, e.g., Peano, on which see E. Landau, *Grundlagen der Analysis*, reprint, New York. 1946; or the discussions on the foundations

ever, questionable whether this conception of a philosophic system is admissible.

First, one may doubt whether the term of a system can be applied with justice to the philosophy of St. Thomas or any other of the Schoolmen. To be sure, none of them has created a system comparable to those, say, of Hegel or another philosopher of recent times. It may be that the notion of a "system," in the modern sense, was unknown to the thinkers of the past, and that we have no right to regret the absence of a thoroughgoing systematization in the writings of either Plato, or Aristotle, or Aquinas. It might be that the modern notion of a system could develop only after the certainty had vanished that the mind is able to apprehend the totality of being as it is in itself. A system may be the expression of an attempt to re construct reality in the human mind, to project, as it were, the imperfectly knowable order of reality on the plane of reason, or – as in the futile but nonetheless grandiose enterprise of Hegel – to evolve the whole of reality out of the subjectivity of the "spirit" as it manifests itself in the human mind.

It is perhaps, wrong to apply the criteria of systematic context to philosophies which were ignorant of the notion of a system in the modern sense. On the other hand, the manifest absence of systematic structure does not necessarily show that it cannot be discovered back of the ideas of such a non systematic thinker. But a system is not necessarily one of the types realized in mathematics. It is, there fore, difficult to state which one of the first principles or the "axiomatic" propositions, the validity of which is taken for granted, has the right of precedence over the others. It is customary to view the doctrines of potency and act, and of matter and form as the two fundamental principles in Aristotelian philosophy. But one might consider that the preference for the universal is still more fundamental. Also, it is hardly possible to decide whether the principle of potency act precedes that of matter form, or whether the opposite relation obtains.

I mention this, because Dr. Day, in one passage, feels that St. Thomas is guilty of a *circulus in arguendo,* and because I shall have to return to this question of the primacy of principles later. Concerning, however, the reproach of circularity, one might point out that to assume several

---

of geometry, which were started by the doctrine of Hilbert on "axiomatic thought" on one hand and the notion of "intuitive mathematics" in Brouwer's works on the other.

"axioms" of equal dignity does not entail any such circularity, even if these axioms support one another to a certain extent.

Dr. Day's contention, as the able exponent of Ockham's ideas that he is, claims that the intellect does not know only by way of abstraction, and hence universals, but is also cognizant of particulars by way of intuition. This intuitive knowledge has no need of a mediating *species intelligibiles*; it is immediate, a direct contact of knowing intellect and known object.

If, however, one asks, how intuitive knowledge of any sort, and especially on the part of the intellect, is possible, one does not receive a clearcut answer. Also, it seems difficult to me to under stand what is the precise meaning of immediacy.

One might indeed argue that the same difficulty arises also in re gard to a theory of intellectual knowledge which appeals only to abstraction, and assumes the mediation by means of a *species intelligibilis*. Whether mediate or immediate, the manner by which the intellect becomes cognizant of any object, universal or particular, or the manner by which the object is conveyed to the intellect, remains ultimately mysterious in either of the two theories. Then, the question is not to arrive at a perfect elucidation, but to determine which theory accords best with the observable facts and offers the simplest explanation. (Although one ought to beware of the idea that simplicity is, as such, already an asset; it may well be that reality is in itself too complex as to allow for an adequate rendering in a simple theory.)

The Thomistic conception of intellectual knowledge rests, ac cording to Dr. Day, primarily on the 'axiomatic" supposition that *intellectus est de universalibus, sensus autem de particularibus*. It seems to me, however, that one cannot well attribute to this proposition the rank of an axiom; it is rather dependent on and rests on one of greater generality. The latter is the principle that there must exist some connaturality between any agent and that acted upon. *Omne ens agit sibi simile*. Which reads, when applied to cognition: *similia similibus cognoscuntur*. This principle can be traced back to Empedocles with whom it appears in the still rather crude form, that man knows the element "earth" and the things consisting of it in virtue of the earthly parts of his being, and so also with the other three elements. The special reference to the elements can be abandoned; the notion relevant here is that some such connaturality has to exist for rendering possible any "affection" of a mental power by an object.

It is here irrelevant whether the principle of individuation is seen in matter, or in the *forma haecceitatis*, or whether individuation is rejected altogether, the particular being envisioned as the only existent and the problem viewed rather as that of generalization or production of the universal. The only relevant point is that the particular things we encounter *in statu viae* are material things, and that to know them as they are we have to know them in their materiality. Hence, in virtue of the principle referred to above, these things can be known only by a power which is itself material or, at least, somehow implies materiality. Materiality can be known only by materiality; and without knowing of its materiality we would not know the thing at all. The principle: *intellectus est de universalibus*, etc., is not a primary supposition, but derived from the principle of connaturality. So far as the notion of intellectual knowledge of universals and the sensory knowledge of particulars is concerned, the reproach of a circular reasoning seems therefore unfounded.

That the material thing is apprehended in the fullness and concreteness of its being by the senses is no point of controversy. The disagreement consists in whether this sensory knowledge of particulars is an exclusive property of the senses, or is shared also by the intellect.

It seems that the intellect has to know about particulars. But it is possible to question that it has to know particulars; knowing about and knowing is not the same thing. I shall try to show that it is not necessary for an explanation of certain intellectual performances to assume that the intellect knows particulars and knows them more or less in the same manner as the senses.

The senses know (or the mind knows in virtue of sensory operations) the particular thing in the concreteness of the thing's being, that is, with all knowable accidental properties and in its materiality,

It is doubtful whether the notion of a *forma haecceitatis*, as individualizing principle, can obviate the difficulties the assumption of a complete and concrete knowledge of particulars encounters when credited to the intellect. This form may well furnish a knowledge of particularity, singularity of the thing, but it is not easy to see how it can be a basis of a knowledge of materiality. This point need not be studied here, however, because knowledge of forms, whether specific or individual, has to be by way of abstraction, and the controversial theory denies the necessity of abstraction and claims an immediate, intuitive knowledge on the part of the intellect.

As has been remarked before, this theory discards the *species intelligibilis* altogether. The intellect is supposed to reach out to the object, or the object is supposed to be present to the intellect without the mediation of any species. What the nature of this immediacy is, remains obscure.

Sensory cognition depends evidently on some demonstrable modification of the organism taking place; this modification is said to be a psychophysical change, because objectively there are alterations in the sense organs and the nervous apparatus connected with them, and because subjectively we are aware of something "happening" to us; there is no doubt that we experience the sensible object as affecting our mind, as intruding into it, as exercising some sort of activity of which we are the more or less passive terminus ad quem. Since the sensed object is not directly "in touch" with the receptive organs, a mediation between the former and the latter is necessary.[6]

This mediation is effected by the impact of physical energy on the sense organ. The existence of bodily changes in the receptory organs is an assured fact of physiology; it has been evident already before experimental analysis became possible. Today, we know much about these changes and are able to follow them from the peripheral organ into the nervous cortical centers. Whatever the relation of these nervous apparatus to our conscious awareness of the thing, it is clear that it is not the latter which reaches these centers and by their alteration enables the mind to become cognizant of the thing; what reaches the centers has no "likeness" to the object, but stand to it in a one to one correlation.[7]

---

6 Even in the case of "touch" there is no direct contact of the sensed object and the receptory organ, and what actually releases tactual sensation is not the object itself, but the deformation of the skin resulting from pressure. Likewise, warmth and cold are not sensed by the warm or cold object contacting the organs of thermaesthesia, but by the flow of warmth from or towards these end organs through the skin.

7 We might make use of a notion which has been suggested by W. Koehler in a different context. Koehler, to build a physiological theory of Gestalt awareness assumes an "isomorphism" of the configurated object on one hand and the distribution of cortical changes on the other. It is not here the question whether this notion achieves what its inventor supposes. Nor need we accept it in just the same sense as it is conceived. But we may well

It is a mistake to believe that the "image" created in the sensory apparatus has to be understood as a "portrait" of the object. This misleading interpretation is suggested by certain vivid memory images, be it of sight or of hearing. But there are many such memory images which are very incomplete, show no physical similarity whatsoever with the object they "represent," and are nonetheless perfectly sufficient for letting the mind deal with things not actually present.

The mind is not conscious of these bodily alterations; it does not know of the processes going on in the retina of the eye or the organ of corti in the ear. It is not more conscious of the processes released in the centers. These bodily changes are truly the *id quo* and not the *id quod* which is known. They mediate somehow between the *res extra* and our knowledge thereof. As far as I can see, there is no fundamental difference between the Thomistic theory of sensory awareness and that based on the results of modern experimental investigation. The one can be translated into the other.

Sensory awareness is envisioned as the prototype of intuitive knowledge. Through the senses we know of the self presence of a thing. The term intuition itself is taken from sense experience. The senses tell us – under average conditions – that a concrete thing is self present and presented: this is the essence of intuitive cognition.

There can be, therefore, no incompatibility of intuitive knowledge on one hand and mediation of such knowledge on the other. In other words, if it were possible provided one had sufficient reasons therefore to maintain the existence of intellectual intuition and nonetheless, at the same time, admit some sort of mediation, that is the efficacy of a species. This seems to have been, at least implicitly, the idea of some medieval "Realists" when they draw a parallel be tween sensory cognition of particulars and intellectual cognition of universals. As the senses intuit the former, so the intellect the latter, which are conceived as existent realities. But we are not concerned here with the question of an intuitive knowledge of universals nor with that of their ontological status.

---

speak of an isomorphism between the object, the changes wrought by the physical energy emanating from the object in the sense organ first, in the nervous apparatus then. I have explained on other occasions that this is precisely the meaning of *imago* and *similitudo* as the Scholastics understand these terms.

It seems inevitable that one assume some link in between the particular and the knowing power, whether this be sensory or intellectual. Neither here nor there can the object be as such present in the knowing power. It must be somehow "represented"; something has to take the object's place in the cognitive context, so that this context and the thing therein become a true *similitudo* of reality. To be present or presented to a mental power is not the same thing as to be present in this power.

We are not conscious of such a "representative" of the thing (or, for that matter of any other content of intellectual knowledge); we know only the thing or, generally speaking, the "object" of our intellectual performance. Nonetheless, the existence of such a "re presentative" must be postulated. This something mediates between the trans subjective datum and the cognitive awareness thereof. It is truly the *id quo* we know; it is never the *id quod*. Insofar there is a strict analogy of sensory and intellectual cognition. This analogy is not suggested, as some think, by a desire for "symmetry" or systematic architectonics; it is imposed by the facts themselves.

If the foregoing reasoning is correct, and one must assume some sort of mediation for sensory as well as for intellectual knowledge in any case, the question arises what the nature of such a mediation might be which establishes a relation between the intellect and the particular. One has to bear in mind as I pointed out before, that to "know" the particular implies that it be presented to the knowing power in the fullness of its being, that is, in its materiality.

The mediation between particular known and knowing intellect cannot be of the same kind as on the level of sensory cognition, This would amount to an incomprehensible duplication of cognitive performances, and also entail that the same effect – namely the intuitable self presence of the object – would result in two powers which *per definitionem*[8] differ from one another. Since the effect of an agent depends on the agent and on that on which it acts, the difference of intellect and sense renders an identity of effect impossible. Therefore,

8 *Per definitionem*: since the intellect is credited with the capacity of abstraction and generally viewed as "higher" than the sense, the difference is acknowledged. If it were not, the reference by Dr. Day to the need of attributing to the intellect *eminentius* what the lower power can achieve, would become meaningless.

any identification of sensible and intellectual species becomes likewise impossible.

From the preceding discussion one can, I believe, conclude that there has to be (1) a mediating something establishing the relation of cognition between knowing intellect and known object not less necessarily than on the level of sensory cognition, and that this mediating something might as well be named a *species intelligibilis*; (2) that this species cannot be the same, either numerically or generically, in both instances.

But how is one to conceive of such a mediation between the material particular and the intellect? All influence the former can exercise on the organism is necessarily also of the material order; it is physical energy and the transformation wrought by it in the bodily sense organs. I see no way by which an affection of the intellect by the material object can be imagined.

The human organism, however, is a psychophysical being; the union of mind and body allows for a simultaneous affection of the bodily organs and of the mental powers. Reference to this has been made before; the *species sensibilis impressa* is a psychophysical alteration. The only possibility of establishing a relation of the res extra and the intellect is through the mediation of those changes wrought by the impact of energy first and "expressed" in the sensory power then, as the percept and the corresponding phantasm.[9]

But the phantasm too is material, even if less so than the thing in reality. The product of sensory performances cannot enter more into the intellect than the material thing. The difficulties the idea of intellectual intuition encounters are the same were one to try to make the intuited object the phantasm. Of these difficulties I have spoken to some extent in an article published some years ago. I need not take up this question again.

But then, the only way out seems to be the assumption that something "happens" to the thing as it presented or represented in the mind, or rather within the whole human being. What happens to the *species sensibilis expressa*, the percept or the phantasm, is described in

9 It would need too long a discussion were I to refer to the notion of an abstractive activity on the sensory level. It is not to be denied that the partial "stripping" of material conditions or the relative dematerialization of the thing, when the phantasm is formed, is in a way an analogy to abstraction *sensu stricto*. But it is not more than an analogy.

a manner too well known to be described here again, by the theory of abstraction, the function of the *intellectus agens*, and so on.

This theory stands, of course, not by itself; it is most closely re to various tenets of Thomistic philosophy. When it is asserted that the product of abstractive activity is the universal, it is presupposed that something like a universal nature is rightly assumed. It is also presupposed that this universal nature is in a certain sense separable from the particular being in which it resides, separable obviously not on the level of the res extra, but of the representatives of these as they emerge from the process of sensory cognition by which the knowing mind "makes its own," as it were, the object whose existential concreteness never can enter into or become part of the mind.

One can conceive of other theories, especially if one abandons the principle of an essential difference between rational and sub rational powers. If one places oneself on the standpoint of many contemporary psychologists and assumes that there is a continuity, first from the merely sensory forms of awareness to the conceptual operations, and second, that there is correspondingly a continuity from animal to human organization, including the mental powers, then one may easily affirm that there is neither any fundamental difference of sensory cognition of the particular and intellectual cognition of either the particular or the universal. The whole difference, then, dwindles to one of looking at the same object under varying angles, and it may be described as an effect of attention. One time, I focus on the thing in its concrete wholeness, another time on a partial aspect, e.g., its color, a third time on what it shares of properties with other things.[10] Such a view can be maintained, if one abandons the idea that the universal is something, in one sense or the other. Nominalism, in one of its shades, leads ultimately to such views. I am afraid that the blurring of the differences between intellectual, rational performances, *actus humani*,

10 It should be noted that, in virtue of such implicit notions, some psychologists use the term "abstraction" in a sense rather different from that usual Thomism or in Scholasticism in general. They name abstraction any mental process, by which a partial aspect is made object of mental activity. Thus, they speak of an "abstraction of similarity," referring to the awareness of likeness in various presented objects under conditions (e.g., very short time of exposure) which do not allow for an adequate apprehension of all features of the objects. It were false to criticize these men for misunderstanding the nature of abstraction; they simply speak of a different set of facts.

and those which are common to man and animal, *actus hominis*, and all the consequences resulting from such failure to discriminate, can be obviated only if at least a minimum of realism, in the medieval sense, is retained. Because of such consequences, many of which have actually resulted in the history of ideas, I believe that all efforts ought to be made for upholding this minimum of realism.

Dr. Day generously recognizes that I have not tried to diminish the difficulties inherent in the Thomistic notion of the intellectual knowledge of particulars. I have attempted to indicate a solution, differing somewhat from that usually proposed, without giving up the basic principles of Thomistic philosophy. It seemed to me that there is no need for the intellect to know the particular in precisely the same manner as the sensory powers know it, because another sort of knowledge apparently suffices to enable the intellect to per- form all the acts proper to this power.

The suggested solution appeals to the curious and not yet sufficiently studied of awareness of "boundaries," There is no problem in knowing the boundaries between two equally known things or classes as such. But the problem arises in its gravity the moment we consider it under the angle implied, for instance, in the question raised by Kant: what are the boundaries of human reason? How can reason determine its own boundaries without, at the same time, transcending them and laying hands, as it were, on the unknowable? When Kant speaks, in the Prolegomena, of the "thing in itself" as a "limit notion" of reason, he implies that reason has some capacity to look beyond its own boundaries. I have referred to Nic. Hartmann's remark that the "transintelligible must possess a minimum of intelligibility," because otherwise we could not speak, let alone conceive of it. But it cannot be denied that to refer to the transintelligible is a meaningful statement. The study of Dr. Day offers a welcome opportunity to return to this subject.[11]

First, I have to submit a question, which at first sight may seem rather shocking because it assumes the questionability of a position which is, so far as I can see, generally taken for granted. But it behoves the philosopher to envision as potentially questionable also, and even

11 Although I have not changed my views on this point, one will easily under stand that they appear to me today in a somewhat different light. And I believe that I have made a little progress towards the elucidation of this obscure question.

particularly, the things which are taken for granted, thought obvious, or labelled self evident. One has always to bear in mind that we may take for granted things without cogent reasons and view them as evident, although they are anything but that; they are only things to which we are accustomed; they are "obvious" only in the sense that we come across them continuously, and therefore neglect to inquire into the *quaestio iuris* as well as the *quaestio facti*.

I ask: Is it true that the intellect knows the particular as such and in such a manner that its knowledge becomes comparable to that of the senses? Is the intellectual knowledge of the particular a knowledge of it in its concreteness and the fullness of its being?

The main reason for taking for granted this sort of intellectual knowledge seems to be the fact that our mind forms judgments of which the grammatical subject is a particular: Socrates is a man; this thing there is a cat. It is supposed that the intellect to arrive at such a proposition must have present both the particular subject and the universal predicate. Hence, the intellect has to know the particular, and must possess a knowledge thereof more or less of the same nature as the knowledge the senses have, because otherwise the intellect could not refer to an actually present thing (this thing there). In such an instance, it seems, the intellectual knowledge must comprise the object (particular) in the fullness and concreteness of the latter's existence. If, however, I form a judgment on Socrates, who is not present *hic et nunc*, the knowledge of the particular might be, if one may say so, an attenuated one, distant and different from that of the senses, when these are placed face to face with the living man Socrates. The mental operation, by which I now think the proposition concerning Socrates need not be the same as it was in the mind of an Athenian contemporary of the sage, encountering him on the streets of his city. One might argue, however, that this difference in the manner of intellectual knowledge (in the case of Socrates as set over against "this thing there") is merely apparent and resulting from the simple fact that our knowledge of Socrates is rather poor. It will be, however, more to the point if another pair of intellectual performances is considered.

Seeing the cat, I say: This thing is a cat. But I may think thing of the cat also when the animal is not present. I talk to someone about my cat; then what I mean is rendered (although never expressed in so complete and so complicated a manner) by: The thing I could point out to you, were you to come home with me, and which I now recall, is a cat. I cannot discover any difference in the intellectual or judgmental operations in these two instances. All the difference that exists, is not in the intellect or its operations but in the total mental situation as it develops in the one and in the other case. I believe that one may perfectly distinguish between what I may call for the moment the sensory (perceptual, respectively imaginative) component and the intellectual judgmental operation. The difference, then, is not in the latter but founded on the introspective evidence that perceiving and imagining are two distinct operations. Everybody knows that there is a great difference between "intuiting" a thing in its self presence and re presenting it by means of an however well developed memory image. The judgment of the intellect can be founded on either the percept or the image; but it is not necessary that the percept be perfectly clear, nor that the image be a true "portrait" or "copy" of the thing. In many people, the imaginative power is rather poor; they are unable to visualize things not present or to recall, with some degree of clarity, auditory phenomena. Nonetheless, their judgments on things absent is not less correct than that of those whose imagination presents them with fully developed images. Even in the case of people who dispose of an effective imaginative power, the highly developed ("photo graphic") images are not the rule; often these images are fleeting, fugitive, ghost like appearances, which, however, suffice for a basis of judgments and even for, what subjectively, is a perfect recalling of a thing once experienced. Our memorative knowledge comprises much more than is given in the image itself.

Be it noted that no intuitive knowledge on the part of the intellect is needed for rendering this power aware of its judging on objects present or absent. For this knowledge it suffices that the mind be conscious of the differences of perceptual and memorative activities.[12]

12 It is not the content, the richness in details, the colorfulness or any such quality which distinguishes the image from the percept. The difference is wholly on the side of the mental performance and its peculiarities, on the side of what Brentano Husserl called "acts" or Stumpf opposed to the "phenomena" (*Erscheinungen*) as "functions," A confusion of image and precept occurs, under average condition, very rarely if at all. It happens that one may not be quite sure whether one perceives or imagines in the case of incomplete sensory data; in such a case one may say I am not sure whether I really see this or that or only imagine it. But this hap pens because there are certain vague visual data and one is not certain whether the interpretation given to them is correct or not. A true confusion of image and percept can

The judgment as such is independent of the self presence of the thing. I may form evident judgments also on pure figments of the mind; if I create in my imagination a fabulous animal, a winged horse for instance, I can make true statements on this creature. Sensory intuition, as it is the characteristic of the external senses, is not necessary. And the evidence the intellect has of judging on a real or a fictitious being depends neither on such an intuition, but on the peculiarities of the total mental situation in perceiving on one hand, and imagining on the other.

St. Thomas does not claim, as I have pointed our in one of the previous studies, that the peculiar operation he calls *reflexio super phantasma* is a necessary factor in the intellectual performance of judging. He rather is of the opinion that a judgment on particulars (Socrates is a man) results from the co operation of the *ratio particularis* with the intellect; if this is the case, no intellectual knowledge of the particular or intuition of it is demanded, because the *ratio particularis s.vis cogitativa* is able, being one of the internal senses, to avail itself directly of the percept or phantasm.[13]

One might argue that the intellect has, all the foregoing remarks notwithstanding, to know immediately the particular because otherwise there can be no evidence of truth or falsehood of a judgment. Truth is the *adaequatio intellectus ad rem. Intellectus* means, I suppose,

---

be brought about under quite unusual experimental conditions; normally how ever, an image even if very vivid and complete is not taken for the presence of a thing. This should be considered before one credits the pathological fact of hallucination with any relevance in regard to the question of perception and imagination. In, truth, hallucinations are mostly not at all what psychiatrists believed them to be, namely particularly vivid images which, in virtue of their "portrait likeness" resemble perfectly perceptions. Quite to the contrary, true hallucinations are very imperfect data, and it is only the interpretation given to them by the diseased mind which makes them into realities. The argument taken from hallucinations, be it in regard to the questions referred to here, be it in regard to the epistemological question of the trustworthiness of our perceptions, should be dropped altogether. It is rather remarkable that the same philosophers who are so extremely distrustful of the testimonies of common sense take at their face value the statements of mentality ill people.

13 This problem need not be discussed here because I am concerned only with the alleged necessity to assume an intellectual intuition of particulars.

in this context not the mental power but its "product"; in this sense *intellectus* is synonymous to concept, when such one is viewed in itself, and to the "state of affairs" expressed in a proposition, when the concept is envisioned as related to another or to a particular. The *res*, in regard to a judgment or proposition, is a relation and thus an object in a sense somewhat different from that in which a particular thing is given this name.[14] An insight into the correspondence of a state of affairs, among real things, particulars, and the relation established in the intellect apparently renders inevitable that this power have direct access to the particular, insofar as this is one member of the relation stated. Suppose, I have a cat called Socrates; then the proposition: Socrates is a cat, will appear as true. But it can appear thus only if the intellect knows of the cat called Socrates. This reasoning, however, is not as cogent as it seems at first sight. For the intellect to know that the proposition is true, it would suffice that one be intellectually aware of the fact that there is "a" cat called Socrates, i.e., that it is legitimate to combine the two names.

The mere awareness that a thing is self present, therefore perceived, or represented, therefore imagined, may exist without any participation of the intellect. Although it is true that language is an achievement closely linked up with rationality, since no sub human being possesses language in the true sense of the name, it does not follow that all verbal utterances are necessarily based on intellectual operations. The so called judgment of existence, of the form: There is this thing, is probably made without co operation of the intellect, as long as the predication of a class name is omitted.[15]

---

14 A. v. Meinong, accordingly, has suggested that one ought to use different names for the res with which the different mental performances, respectively the powers are concerned. He calls "object" the "referent" of sensory activities (including imagination), but an "objective" (*das Objektiv*) the state of affairs expressed in a judgment.

15 The mind is not forced to proceed from sensory awareness to the formation of a universal. It may stay on the level of mere sensory awareness. We may "be lost in the contemplation" of a thing without going on to classification or generalization. Usually, the habit of naming and therewith of generalization and abstraction prevails. But there are cases in which we are so captivated by sensory impressions that we abandon ourselves to them without "thinking" at all, e.g., when listening to enthralling music. One can train oneself to forget about intellectual co-operation and learn to live, as it were, on the level of unadulterated sensuality, Perhaps, I may make use of

When we, as it is generally the case, immediately apply a general name to a particular sensed or imagined, the intellect seems to have to be cognizant of this particular. This must be so, it is claimed, because otherwise the suitability of the general name and the concept it designates could never be ascertained. It is here again where the controversial *reflexio super phantasma* comes in. According to the theory criticized by Dr. Day, the intellect possesses only an abstract knowledge of "the man," "the cat" in general. St. Thomas says, as one knows, that the intellect becomes cognizant of the reference its general concept has to a given particular by the intellect retracing its steps and finally discovering the particular phantasm as the origin of the whole abstractive and conceptual process.

I believe that to arrive at a further clarification of this point one has to take account of certain facts and ideas which, I dare say, are not sufficiently considered by psychology.[16] One has to assume that in virtue of the correlation between mental operation and the objects with which this operation is concerned or to which it refers, each act of a power is differentiated by its object. Although perceiving is always fundamentally the same sort of operation, to perceive colors is not the same as to perceive sounds; and to perceive colors is neither the same as to perceive shape or distance. Likewise intellectual operations differ according to the objects with which they deal or the region in which they move; thus, it is not the same kind of thinking when a mind is

---

this opportunity to warn against the belief that introspection is easy and to be achieved by everyone. Like all other procedures, introspection too must be trained to be reliable. Many mistakes have arisen by the confidence untrained observers placed in their, often casual, observations. Also, it is absolutely imperative that introspective evidence be collected from a greater number of observers, in view of the manifold individual differences of which one cannot say beforehand how and to what an extent they modify inner experience.

16 Modern psychology, that is. If such things as those I am going to discuss are not mentioned in medieval texts, one has to realize that descriptive psychology was not a primary concern with the writers of these centuries. However acute their observations are, they are used mainly as illustrations and empirical proofs of this or that philosophical doctrine. Description for description's sake would probably appear to the medieval thinkers as an idle occupation. There are many problems which did not arise within the context of medieval reflection. But since they arise today, it is our duty to consider carefully all available evidence.

preoccupied with a problem of mathematics or with one of another kind.[17] There is, in medieval psychology, one or the other notion which seems to indicate that the thinkers of this age were not unaware of these facts; the notion of the practical intellect is one of them, as is also the characterization of prudence as *recta ratio agendi* as set over against the *recta ratio faciendi,* called science.

The shading or coloring of mental acts by their respective objects becomes more visible when one turns from simple performances, as the awareness of shape or distance, or also thinking about this or that matter, to a consideration of the total response on the part of a person to the total situation in which he is engaged. If Fichte's much quoted word affirms that it depends on what a man is, what kind of philosophy he has, it is also true that the kind of philosophy one has fashions, to a notable degree, the manner of one's being. Not only depends the world view on personal peculiarities, but the opposite relation obtains too. One can base a typology on the various ways of looking at reality as one can correlate these views with mental types.

Once, chiefly by a study of the "worlds" different persons possess, one's attention has been aroused, one discovers that there is an enormous wealth of shades within the performances of one and the same mental power. These powers are distinguishable not only *secundum operationes et objecta,* but the single operations of one power are likewise shaded by the objects to which they refer.[18]

Modern philosophical speculation and psychological inquiry have paid but little attention to these facts. One reason may be that observation is not quite easy, and that the possibility of such differentiations must be suspected, perhaps, first before one can discover them. Another reason, however, is probably more influential. The modern

17 Particularly, it is one thing to think in purely "symbolic" terms, as in mathematics, and in terms possessing real significance. It is because of the neglect of these facts that the erroneous idea developed that a training in mathematics and science amounts to a training of the intellect as a whole. If there is such a generally effective training, it is probably rather that attained by grammar and languages than that by learning how to operate symbols.

18 One might consider, in this context, the ideas of C. Spearman on the nature of human intellect. He assumes that there is a "general factor, called g, which determines the over all ability of a person's intellect, and that it is determined more particularly by a number of additional special factors, s1, s2, ...

mind, even that of Neo-Scholastics, has suffered the permeation of all modern thought by the philosophy of Descartes.

Even a man who consciously rejects the tenets of Cartesianism cannot help, unless he is particularly attentive, falling under this influence. Psychology, especially, however much, the individual psychologist may be sure that no philosophical prejudice determines his attitude, has suffered this influence ever since its birth about a century ago. The Cartesian *cogito* emphasizes exclusively, if one applies it to psychological problems, the subjective aspect; the *cogitatio* alone is important. Descartes ignored the unsolvable connection between the *cogitatio* and the *cogitatum*. Critical philosophy, developing in the wake of Cartesianism, contributed still more to this emphasis. It is about time that psychology free itself from the allegiance to this philosophy.[19]

In consequence of this strict correlation of mental act and object it is impossible to attribute to two different operations the same object. One and the same object cannot be known in the same manner by two different powers. To claim, therefore, that the intellect, as a power of greater dignity, must be capable of the same achievements as the senses besides those which are proper to the rational power alone, appears to me as a statement not only lacking foundation in fact but as one flatly contradicting the facts.[20]

Even if one were to admit that there exists some sort of intuitive ability in regard to particulars in the intellect, the effect of this intuition cannot possibly be the same as it is on the level of sensory performance. But the senses apprehend the particular in the concreteness and plenitude of its being, as *hic et nunc et tale*. What then is left to the intellect to know of the particular?

It is, I submit, not necessary that the intellect know the particular ut sic. The intellect deals with the particular when applying to it a general notion; it has to be certain that the concept fits to the particular. This

---

19 It is not uninteresting to observe that the recent attempt of Husserl to take account of the objective aspect ends after all in an idealistic philosophy. Cf. S. Vanni Rovighi, *La Filosofia di Edmund Husserl*, Milan, 1939.

20 I have carefully and intentionally avoided quoting any passage in Aquinas I might use as a confirmation of my views. As long as it is feasible to plead for one's ideas by referring to facts, one should not shelter behind "authorities," *Auctoritas autem habet cereum nasum, qui in quamlibet potest flecti directionem*; this warning by Alanus ab Insulis should not be forgotten.

necessity arises first when a new particular of the same species comes under observation and is recognized as "one more instance;" secondly, when a universal is predicated of a particular.

In the first case, no intuitive knowledge is necessary. If the intellect proceeds to abstract a universal from the newly encountered instance, it may identify this with the universal abstracted previously[21] without any immediate intuitive contact between mental power and particular object. In the other case, it seems sufficient that the intellect be aware of the "total mental situation," that is, of the state in which the sensory cognitive powers are and to be able to identify this state with that having occurred previously when the universal was formed by way of abstraction. Here, neither, can I see a need for appealing to an immediate intellectual intuition.

In an article published several years ago I pointed out that the image or phantasm which is necessarily re presented when the intellect returns to a concept formed before, need not at all be the very same phantasm as the one from which the universal had been abstractively derived. What is needed is simply some act of the imaginative power, not however the reproduction of the very same image. In fact, the images which "stand for" a perceived object can vary in every instance of reproduction; divers images may function as representatives of the same object; the images may be "life like" or fragmentary or even symbolic, so that the phenomenon shows no similarity with the original object.

---

21 Sometimes things are described as if the intellect were forced to abstract a universal whenever the knowing mind is cognizant of an object. This is obviously untrue. I have pointed out above that the mind may stay on the level of purely sensory awareness without proceeding to either generalization or abstraction. (Not all generalization is abstractive; there is also a generalization by way of a general image; this is for instance, the basis of "schematic" drawings, as they may be found in many textbooks; the "characteristic features," say, of the gothic architecture in a history of fine arts are not reproductions of individual windows or spires, but "imaginative generalizations" or "general images,") Another error which occurs frequently is to assume that abstraction demands a collection of similar items; but it is not only in principle possible to abstract the universal nature of a newly encountered thing if it comes under observation only once and in one single instance, it is also certain that in some cases such abstraction is achieved under such conditions; it suffices to have seen one triangle to know the universal nature of triangularity.

It is much more the rule that the phantasm reproduced in such situations be utterly unlike the object than that it possess a "portrait" quality. However mysterious this may be, it is nonetheless certain that these strange, incomplete images fulfill perfectly the task to represent the object. But then, it becomes impossible to speak of an intuition on the part of the intellect by which this power would be brought in immediate contact with the object.[22]

I do not and cannot claim to have answered all the objections raised by Dr. Day. Neither can I pretend at having presented here an exhaustive survey of either problems or facts. Both tasks are too big for the space reasonably allowed to an article. Such as it stands, my argument justifies, I believe, certain conclusions which may be summarized in a few words.

1. The empirical evidence in favor of an intuitive knowledge of particulars on the part of the intellect is insufficient and, insofar as it exists, not in favor of the thesis.

2. If one were to assume that the intellect knows the particular intuitively in the same concreteness and fullness as is supplied by sensory cognition, this would entail (a) an unnecessary duplication of knowledge (which indeed ought to be repulsive to any follower of Ockham); (b) a neglect of the fundamental and necessary correlation of known object and knowing power; (c) a disregard of observable facts, as they have been briefly indicated in the foregoing pages.

3. The reasons alleged for the necessity of such an intellectual intuitive knowledge are not cogent; the various problems raised can be solved also on the basis of a theory which credits the intellect with abstractive knowledge only.

4. The theory of intellectual intuition encounters at least as many difficulties as that of which I am made, by Dr. Day, the representative and advocate.

---

22 The disregard of introspection as a method of inquiry with the "modern" experimentalists and the lack of training with the Neo-Scholastics has created the rather regrettable situation that obvious problems, very much in need of investigation, are overlooked. But it is important that they be studied; the experimentalist might profit by being made aware of questions he can study with his own methods, and the philosopher might be warned not to envision the data he possesses as complete and as furnishing all the empirical evidence he needs.

I do not, as I have said before, feel entitled to act as a spokesman of the Neo-Thomistic school; I am not at all sure that all Neo-Thomists will approve of my views. But having been thus challenged, I did not consider it right to remain silent. And I repeat, that the procedure I tried to adopt, viz., to present my views in an affirmative form rather than by way of criticism, seemed to me more fruitful and also more worthy of the kindness and acumen of my adversary.

PHILOSOPHIA – PHILANTHROPIA

Philosophy means love of wisdom. Philanthropy means love of man. Is it wise to love man? Does wisdom, or what kind of wisdom does, suggest that man is lovable, and that therefore one ought to love "one's neighbor"? It is not for wisdom to command or compel. Wisdom only counsels, and the wise man is he who heeds. Does wisdom advise that man love his fellows? And if it does, in what sense should this advice be understood?

Suppose that concrete conditions make it imperative that there be friendship and even love among men, and suppose furthermore that several widely different sets of ideas, all claiming to be wisdom, are offered; then one may ask: if such is my and everyone's desire, what ideas may I choose to provide an intelligible basis for my demands? The mere existence of a demand, however general, is not any demonstration of its reasonableness. It might be that man desires everlasting peace, mutual understanding, cooperation, and nonetheless deludes himself, aspiring to what is denied by an inexorable destiny. Such a view has been rejected by all those thinkers with some sort of theistic view; one recalls Descartes's argument of the *deus malignus*. To others it appeared unthinkable that a primary need of human nature should be utterly incapable of fulfilment; as they used to say, *natura non agit superfluum*.

There have been philosophies which were far from commending any sort of neighborly love. Some have considered man hateful. Others have felt that only a few of their fellows deserved love and esteem, whereas the rest appeared contemptible. There were those whose attitude was that of pity rather than of love and who showed consideration for their fellows not on the latter's but on their own behalf – to acquire merit, or because *noblesse oblige*.

But "thou shalt love thy neighbor as thyself," say the Scriptures. And Master Eckhart commented on this: "If you do not love the man you never saw as much as yourself, you are on the wrong way." Of this love speaks the well known chapter in Corinthians I, of the love called agape or caritas, disinterested, "not seeking its own." The idea is that we should love our "neighbor" not for the sake of any gain, either here or hereafter, not because loving him will provide satisfaction to some inclination, nor because of merit we acquire, but because he is a neighbor – in the language of Christian theology, a child of God, actual or potential.

Little knowledge of history is needed to realize that this ideal of love has never been attained by a notable number. But as long as Christian doctrine was universally recognized in the Western world, this ideal stood, at least, as an ultimate directive before man's eyes. Man sinned as much in medieval times as in any other age, but he knew that he sinned and did not embellish his deficiencies by calling them right.

If neighborly love could claim absolute compulsiveness only because of its Divine origin or if no intelligible reason might be discovered for such a demand, then the situation of the world would be hopeless. However, the idea that certain truths, considered as revealed by the faithful, can also be discovered in the "light of natural reason," is stated by the great exponents of theology. Thus, Thomas Aquinas says that Revelation contains many truths which man may also discover by himself; but not all being able to do so, Divine Mercy provided by Revelation for all to know these truths;

I refer to these ideas not to appeal to the authority of a *doctor ecclesiae*, but to point out that even he, who assuredly credited Revelation with the most important role in man's life, admitted the knowability of certain truths also without the intervention of a supernatural power. Even though the notion of one's "neighbor" received its full meaning only after and through the spread of Christianity, it is in no way alien to non-Christian and pre Christian thought![1]

---

1 *Comment by Harry B. Friedgood:*
The essence of the spiritual teachings of Christianity, Judaism, Buddhism, Confucianism, and Mohammedanism is that one cannot jive to or for oneself; that love of one's neighbor is essential to man's happiness and peace of mind and to the fulfilment of his destiny. This is an age old truth which modern psychiatrists have reduced to scientific formulation through the methodology of psychoanalysis.

Freudian psychoanalysis has been accused of being a foe of religion to the extent that it has tampered, in the case of Catholicism, for instance, with the concepts of sin and confession. In my experience, psychoanalysis also has had the effect of reaffirming in some individuals the validity of certain aspects of their religious faith, against which they had reacted unfavorably for unconscious reasons prior to analytic therapy.

It seems, therefore, a legitimate task to inquire into the rational foundation of neighborly love, and hence of "philanthropy." Obviously, it is the task of philosophy to provide such a foundation.

Any such attempt encounters several objections. It is argued that theoretical ideas have no influence on the shaping of man's life or on "practical" questions. Some do not believe in the power of reason to determine human behavior; others think that speculation and theory appear only as an after effect, when the course of history has already brought forth certain events. The latter side with Hegel's well known phrase of Minerva's bird spreading its wings only in the dusk of the evening. But even if the real forces shaping man's life are other than those of reason, nonetheless these forces become effective mainly when they are formulated in an intelligible manner. Ideas, after all, have played a decisive role in history. However much a theory of history like that of Marx may emphasize the basic importance of economic or other social factors, it has to recognize that goals have to be stated, approaches clarified, ideas rendered conscious (e.g., "class consciousness"). It is philosophy which casts into their intelligible forms what is dumbly and vaguely sensed and working without definite direction.

It is furthermore the task of philosophy to point out the problems which are concealed by the things an age or a group takes for granted. The disintegration of certain cherished beliefs, of time honored customs, social structures, political forms, would not strike man with such bewildering force, were he heeding the warnings of philosophy. In Kant's words: the *quaestio iuris* has to be answered, and this answer cannot be anticipated before a careful analysis of the whole set of problems.

It is a general prejudice that single problems may be studied and solved one after the other. That this is true for many practical situations is beyond question. But even in these, one has often to take account of a multiplicity of other problems which, at first sight, seem

In the light of modern experience one cannot regard the tenets of religion and the data of science as mutually exclusive and incompatible. Each has much to learn from the other, if they will but jointly explore their common area of interest, viz., the ultimate significance of life. The welding of faith and fact should relegate the ancient impasse between religion and science to the status of a frayed myth.

As indicated in my paper [Chapter XL, Part I, "The Superego"] the problems involved in ethics, and the truth or falsity of moral ideas, cannot be derided in exclusively psychological terms.

hardly related to the one in the foreground. Such a complicated network of relations is the rule in all "human studies." It is the more so when ultimate questions are considered. If we raise the question, what kind of philosophy might be most suitable as a foundation for philanthropy, we must try to discover the characteristics of such a philosophy as a whole.

True love is only that of persons. All other love, so called, is either mere liking or preference, or it is the result of an unwarranted, maybe even immoral, "personification" (hence we give proper, even human, names to our pets). Another, equally spurious "love" is that we feel for "possessions"; this is mostly self love, and the grief we feel when we have lost one of our possessions is not on behalf of the thing lost, but because we are deprived of it.

The primary condition for brotherly or neighborly love is, accordingly, a sharp distinction between man and any other being. No philosophy which refuses to give to man an unique position in the realm of being can claim to provide a reliable basis of philanthropy.[2]

With the recognition of the uniqueness of human nature must be allied the recognition of the uniqueness of the human person. Things which are interchangeable measure the worth of one another; they therefore "have a price" – but "man alone has dignity." He is in no case interchangeable. Possessing dignity, a peculiar kind of worth or value, he becomes, and only in virtue of this, the goal of the specifically personalistic attitude of love.[3]

---

2 The recognition of the uniqueness of human nature is compatible with all sorts of biological theories; a conception of "emergent evolution" is forced to maintain such an exceptionality of human nature. But other forms of evolutionism may do so as well; the position token by J. Huxley is an example.

3 *Comment by Ralph T. Flewelling:*
The basing of democracy on the uniqueness of man is sound and incontrovertible both politically and psychologically. I like particularly the argument from "uniqueness" as putting man out of the category of "things." Love, too, in the high sense of that term, can exist only where there is potentiality for response, as between human beings.

Comment by Edgar S. Brightman:
The essential point of Doctor Allers's paper – that the love of one's neighbor is rational – is in my judgment thoroughly sound. It is in harmony with Plato, the Stoics, Kant, and modern personalism, as well as with St.

This recognition can be based on intelligible grounds only if there is recognition of an objective order of values. All relativism is by its very nature opposed, in last resort, to the recognition of the peculiar dignity of the human person.[4] As soon as values are made relative to any set of circumstances, be they individual "interest," or social and historical conditions, there is no longer any reason to justify the exceptionality of the human being.

None of the arguments taken from psychology and from cultural anthropology against an absolute and objective order of values proves tenable. It is not true that values are "felt," apprehended on the basis of emotional or appetitive experience; rather these mental states are responses ensuing after an apprehension of value which is in itself of the nature of a cognitive process. Nor is it true that the comparative study of civilization proves a relativity of values. What is true is that the extensiveness of certain evaluations is viewed differently at different cultural stages (e.g., the notion of "neighbor," evolving from the restricted use only in regard to the member of the same tribe through many intermediary stages – of which the *civis Romanus* is a very important one – to our conception which is rooted, at least within Western civilization, in the Christian doctrine). A fargoing relativity exists only in regard to values of a secondary kind and those referring to the lowest class of values, like those of mere sensuous pleasure, as in food. It is already questionable whether esthetic evaluation is as "relative" as it is claimed; maybe we are just be ginning to discover the objective principles of esthetics.

Thomas and St. Paul (especially when one takes the thirteenth and fourteenth chapters of I Corinthians together). It is grounded in the essential nature of persons as persons, while totalitarianism rejects both reason and love. The paper of Doctor Allers is s sound and welcome antidote to current irrationalisms and immoralisms.

4 *Comment by Ralph T. Flewelling;*
The statement seems to me to partake of the fallacy of the universal unless Professor Allers defines his terms more closely. We all believe that an absolute ideal is necessary to the achievement of the highest possible good, but not only will the achievement fall short, but the ideal itself, as conceived, will be transplanted with higher ones as the individual grows morally and spiritually. Values actually achieved are relative to a supreme value, and the comprehension by men of the supreme value is dependent on growing revelations of worth.

It seems the more necessary that the uniqueness and intrinsic dignity of the individual human person be justified on intelligible grounds, because the whole development in recent times tends toward an ever increasing "depersonalization" and "dehumanization" of man. Every situation which forces man into the role of such an indifferent atomic element threatens to deprive him of his dignity; this dignity, being inherent in human nature, never can be actually abolished, but it can be denied utterance and recognition. The more man is viewed mostly as "element" or "member" the less assured he becomes of his personal worth.

Totalitarianism, which represents the height of depersonalizing forces, deprives man totally of his dignity. It is dangerous to make even the slightest concession to this mentality. I am afraid that the distinction some "personalists" make between "person" and "individual" is already too fargoing a step toward the totalitarian conception, however hostile the advocates of this view be to any sort of totalitarianism.[5] It should be noted that totalitarianism is basically a negation; it exists in virtue of the denial of personal worth, thus viewing the person as an instrument subservient to the State, or the Party, or the Race. Totalitarianism does not posit any new view; it draws all its strength from a negation. In this, totalitarianism falls into line with many highly different trends in modern times. It was the pride of philosophy, that affirmations were made on the nature of the universe, on man, his nature and destiny. The thought of the nineteenth century, at least of its second half, felt proud of its negations. The great passion of this century was "debunking," not indeed primarily persons – that was a later product – but everything labelled "higher" in the past. "Reductionism," as this attitude has been called, destroys the manifoldness of reality;

5 *Comment by Ralph T. Flewelling:*
I would like Professor Allers in be more specific, since I myself may be a guilty party. Surely it is allowable, if one defines his terms, to use a term in the sense defined. Individuality might for purposes of discussion be applied to those expressions of the self which separate a man from his fellows, his duties, and she service of God. Individualism might be a mere expression of differences, of oddity, as in the case of flaming neckties and long hair, things by which the individual draws attention to his egotism. Personality also, might be seen as an achievement of the highest self expression which can come only when the individual surrenders his selfish interests to the service of others, loses himself in the spiritual side of his work and the service of God.

its slogan reads: nothing other than ... To a reductionist mentality all "higher" things appear as having fraudulently appropriated this name. In recent days one notices a definite change in this regard, but the leveling down tendency has grown roots in many minds.[6]

I have attempted to show on a previous occasion that the idea of founding neighborly love on "biological facts" is self contradictory and leads to impossible consequences. The same is, so far as I can see, true of all so called naturalistic conceptions which want to give man his due and nonetheless to consider him as a mere "object of nature."[7]

A philosophy which refuses to base its ethical proposals on a general metaphysics and on principles considered as unshakable and of universal validity must prove ultimately unsatisfactory. It cannot answer the *quaestio iuris*. This applies, among other conceptions, to that of utilitarianism. This philosophy, however much it may appeal to many because of its "common sense," has no answer (as long as at remains strictly within its own boundaries) to the objection that there is no intelligible reason why the "greatest happiness of the greatest number" should be made an universally recognized goal. It can be and has been argued that the unhappiness of the many is not too high a price to pay for the happiness of the few who represent some elect, superior group. Nor can utilitarianism define the kind of happiness which man ought to desire and to attain.[8]

---

6 How far the influence goes of this destruction of higher values may be evidenced, e.g., by the remark of a college student in a recent survey. This man, obviously a typical representative of his class, named three things he considered necessary: a reasonably high and secure income, opportunity for sexual satisfaction, opportunity for enjoying life. No word on love, or family, or civic responsibility, or the hope to he useful.

7 The human person can never become an "object" to himself, as has often been said. But strictly speaking neither can he become an object, as other things are, to another. There is no greater degradation of human dignity and human relations than the unfortunate term Freud those to designate the partner in a relation of love: "sexual object."

8 *Comment by David Baumgardt:*
I entirely agree with Professor Allers that secular ethics nerd not be hostile to the essence of the great historic faiths. In his attempt, however, to give us a sketch of a rational ethics Professor Allers is, I think, less successful.
As to his criticism of every type of hedonism, I feel obliged to play the rule of the *advocatus diaboli* at least on two fundamental points. (1) Are the very tame objections Professor Allers makes to utilitarianism not pertinent to

I cannot presume to develop a philosophy that might comply with the indispensable conditions, as I view them, for becoming a reliable foundation of any philanthropic endeavor. I may be allowed, perhaps, to add one concluding remark.

What is the use, some will indubitably ask, of talking of such a philosophy, maybe not even existing, and probably unattainable, if history, past and present, shows so clearly that philosophers have never notably contributed to the fashioning of the real world? I have commented be fore on the fact that this notion of the total inefficacy of philosophy seems to me refuted by the same history to which the critics appeal. Nor should the philosopher be condemned for speaking a language of his own, any more than the scientist is reproved for using formulae and signs which are unknown to the uninitiated. Philosophical ideas have molded the ways of thought of generations without every per-

---

his own ethics? Does not Professor Allers admit himself that "the unshakable" and "universally valid" principles of his own ethics are rejected by the totalitarians in almost the same words as are used against utilitarianism? Certainly, the *quaestio iuris* in ethics cannot be answered by the fact that certain principles are said to be "unshakable" and "universally valid," nor by the other fact that certain people deny the validity of other principles and give some "intelligible reason" for their denial. In astronomy and all other sciences as well as in ethics, the validity of a fundamental principle, i.e., a fundamental hypothesis, can be demonstrated only by the fact that the hypothesis in question presents all the relevant phenomena in a more coherent whole than any other hypothesis. The belief in absolutely valid principles, however, seems in me possible only in theology but not in any science – be it astronomy or ethics.

(2) It seems to me that it is far more hopeful to describe "the kind of happiness which man ought to desire" unambiguously than to describe precisely in what sense a human personality can legitimately be considered as a "member" of the Church and other communities or is illegitimately considered as "a mere element" of those communities: for, utilitarianism ultimately refers so objective facts, the real feelings of man. Professor Allers's ethics, however, refer to concepts which applied to reality may allow rasher different and even contradictory definitions. No Nazi and no Fascist maintained and could maintain that he cared for the "greatest happiness of the greatest number." But many Nazis and Fascists denied and could deny that they "depersonalized" man and treated him as a "mere dement." They even said and, I think, could say that they respected the "dignity" of an opponent by killing him, in the same sense as non totalitarian states respect this dignity even when they execute a criminal.

son being able to under stand perfectly, or at all, what the philosopher said.

The philosopher cannot rule the world. Even Plato realized that his Republic was an utopian construction, as evidenced by his change of attitude in the Laws. The philosopher often has been, and perhaps ought to be more conscious of this, a prophet – one of those who "prepare the way and straighten out the paths."

Minerva's bird, in fact, spreads its wings not only in the dusk of the evening; its flight continues throughout the hours of darkness into the early dawn of a new day.

ETHICS AND ANTHROPOLOGY*

If one were to define ethics broadly enough to include all kinds of moral philosophy, one might submit that ethics is the science of those principles by the application of which man is enabled to arrange his conduct so as to attain his end and fulfill his destiny. It is the view one has of the end and the destiny which determines the particular system of moral philosophy he adopts.

Because dealing with principles, this science is essentially philosophic. This is true even of those ideas on ethics which deny the existence of immutable principles, and hold that ethical doctrines or the moral code change with the changing historical, cultural, or social conditions. Such a relativistic or naturalistic theory is under the obligation to state the general principle which governs the alleged transformations of morals, and requires, therefore, a philosophy of history and civilization as its basis.

A mere description of the moral ideas prevalent at a certain time and in a certain place is not a work of ethics. It may pertain to the history of morals, or form a chapter in cultural anthropology. It is, however, an indispensable work even for a moral philosophy which believes in immutable principles. Such a philosophy may be labeled "dogmatic," with more or less justice; however dogmatic it be, it cannot dispense with the knowledge of empirical facts.

The task of a science of ethics is not, in fact, restricted to statements on principle with, perhaps, some additional remarks of casuistic nature. Account must be rendered of the fact that there are and have been widely different conceptions of morality, and it must be explained why it happens that men diverge so much on such questions.

More important is it that ethics implies the application of the principles it exposes. It has, therefore, to consider the factual situations in which men exist and the factors which determine or modify this application. The situations and factors are either those of an individual, taken in isolation and viewed only insofar as his idiosyncrasies, opportunities, intelligence, and so forth become influential; or one has to

Paper read at the meeting of the District of Columbia Maryland Conference of the American Catholic Philosophical Association, December 2, 1949.

deal with the situations and factors to which a whole group, a people, a nation, is subjected at a certain time and in a certain place.

Thus it becomes necessary that ethics be concerned with an analysis of the circumstances of human existence. Without such an analysis, ethics is bound to be a bloodless, abstract, unappealing collection of propositions.

Ethics is placed, indeed, "between" speculative philosophy on one hand and empirical anthropology on the other. Its in-betweenness is of a peculiar kind, unlike that of other philosophical disciplines.

Cosmology, for instance, is also placed between speculation and empirical knowledge; the former needs to consider the factual evidence the latter provides. Another kind of in-betweenness is that of philosophical psychology which depends on one hand on the principles of metaphysics, on the other on the facts observation and experiment furnish. Part of this evidence is easily found and does not necessitate any particular inquiry; thus it is of common observation that there are cognitive and appetitive performances. But in regard to many other questions careful analysis of facts and a comprehensive knowledge of all the facts available are indispensable, if the speculative psychologist is not to arrive at statements not countenanced, by reality. There is reason to be afraid that philosophical psychology, by not taking sufficient account of observable facts, may one day find itself in a situation comparable to that of the speculative philosophy of nature at the time of Galileo.

One might, perhaps, mention as another philosophical discipline standing in between speculation and observation, that of aesthetics. If aesthetics is conceived of as stating the conditions for the presence or absence of aesthetic values in an object, it becomes a normative science and, at the same time, one concerned with the facts of the history of art, the psychology of artistic or poetic creation, and also with the psychology of aesthetic enjoyment and understanding.

Ethics is viewed, by whatever philosophical school, as being essentially normative. It deals not with human conduct as it actually is, but as it ought to be if it is to he commensurate to man's ends and the fulfillment of his destiny. The note of "oughtness" is characteristic of all systems of ethics, including those of a strictly relativistic nature. At least, for the time being, under the momentarily prevailing circumstances, man ought to behave in this or that manner.

No statement on what man ought to do, no commandment, law, or rule, can be significant, unless account be taken of the capacities of human nature. The often quoted principle of the Roman law is universally true: *Nemo obligetur ultra posse*. Hence, ethics needs to know what are human nature and its abilities in general and how the latter are modified by personal or environmental conditions. Ethics requires a "moral psychology" of which we, unfortunately, as yet know not enough. Since contemporary psychology is not infrequently unwilling to admit anything like will as a distinct power of the mind[1] one need not wonder that there are hardly any studies of the problems related to the exercise of will. This is one point among others, where the determining role of philosophical opinions on empirical research becomes evident. Although. everyone caring to observe his experiences may realize that there is a peculiar state of mind, usually called willing, this observation is simply disregarded, because such a thing as will does not figure in the world picture the psychologist happens to have made his own.

As the psychology of the individual so is the sociology of the group of the greatest importance for the science of ethics. As ethics remains mostly sterile when it loses contact with moral psychology, so it cannot answer a number of its urgent questions if it does not seek information from cultural anthropology.

One may call all sciences dealing with human nature, man as an individual and as a member of the group, anthropology in a wide sense. The concern of ethics with anthropology is, then, twofold. It has a positive aspect, which may be defined as the "justification of ethics by anthropology," and a negative aspect, to be described as the "justification of ethics before anthropology."

The first refers to the demonstration that a given kind of ethics is, if one may say so, commensurate to human nature, that is, that it does not make demands which man cannot meet. This implies the further demonstration of the practicality of the rules laid down by the code of morals under investigation. It has to be shown that the demands ethics makes on man can be fulfilled also under the actually existing conditions.

1 "Will is merely a troublesome word that the psychologist would prefer not to bother the student with. But psychology has inherited it together with many other ambiguous notions, upon which time must be spent, if for no other reason than to demonstrate how little they mean." E. Freeman, *Principles of General Psychology* (New York, 1939), pp. 23 ff.

The other task may be called one of apologetics. In fact, many of the criticisms launched against the Christian code of morals claim to be based on factual evidence supplied by anthropology. This is, of course, a point which needs careful examination.

Nothing deserves more of critical analysis than those statements which purport to be about facts and nothing but facts and which are, in truth, something different. They are reports on "findings" clad in the language of a theory or a philosophy.

It requires not much of analysis to discover that many of the so called factual statements urged against the principles of Christian morality are anything else than simple statements of "facts." They are the outcome of definite philosophical "prejudices" – taking this word in its literal sense without any disparaging connotation – which pertain to the set of ideas known as psychologism, naturalistic "humanism," and relativism.

The criticisms brought forth are first directed against the basic assumption that there are immutable principles of morals which retain their validity whatever the cultural and social situation may be. These criticisms must be met otherwise than by merely reasserting one's own standpoint. Such a procedure does not lead anywhere. It is necessary that the fight be carried into the opponent's own terrain.

The affirmation of immutable principles is based, within a philosophical consideration,[2] on the notion that human nature is the same under all circumstances, in particular that it is the same however widely different the state of civilization may be.

The idea that man's nature is not stable but has changed notably in the course of the thousands of years of his way from the pre-paleolithic age to our times, that between our way of thinking and acting on one hand and that of the primitives there is a profound gap, and therewith the further notion that a man cannot truly understand another if the other is a member of a totally different civilization and, especially, speaks a language of a totally different structure, all these notions had found a powerful support in the theory proposed by the eminent French philosopher and sociologist Lucien Lévy-Bruhl in 1910.

The ideas of Lévy-Bruhl are known well enough as to make any detailed report unnecessary. His main contentions were: that the primitive mind does not operate by means of the principle of contradiction,

2 That is, leaving aside all reference to divine commandments and revealed truth.

that this principle is replaced in the mind of the primitive by the "law of participation," and that the essence of "archaic" mentality, is to be described as "magic thinking." Lévy-Bruhl's ideas were sharply criticized by some outstanding students of cultural anthropology, among whom the late B. Malinovski deserves mention. They were criticized also by a number of psychologists. It was pointed out that the "magic" way of thinking is limited to very definite fields, that the primitive is quite capable of reasoning as we do in all practical questions, that he displays ingenuousness and appears to be sufficiently "logical" to allow him to cope with the situations he encounters.

These criticisms were, however, not able to stem the enthusiastic reception the theory of Lévy-Bruhl was given by a great many psychologists and anthropologists. The reason for this widespread approval was, probably, the close alliance these ideas formed with Freudian psychoanalysis. This doctrine came, as is known, to be almost generally accepted and to be considered as the greatest achievement first in the field of psychology, but soon in all studies concerned with human nature and human affairs.

Freud had conceived of certain abnormal mental states as being caused by what he called regression: that is a return to a developmental stage which the individual has passed and on which he falls back when unable to come to terms with reality. But Freud had introduced in his theory still another idea. He believed that the laws of development as they are seen in the mental growth of the individual are the same as those which govern the development of mankind in the history of civilization. He simply applied the so called principle of ontogenesis to history. This principle, as formulated by Haeckcl, states that individual development recapitulates in a much abbreviated form the history of the race; the fertilized egg cell corresponds thus to the hypothetical unicellular ancestor of all living beings; a later stage corresponds to organisms of a more complex structure; the human embryo passes through a stage reminiscent of the anatomy of fishes, and so forth. Freud assumed that individual mental development likewise recapitulates history, not of the race as a biological unit, but of the series of cultural stages which preceded the time when modern man emerged from the stone age and marched onwards until he reached his present kind of civilization. The infant is still an animal, and the small child has the mentality of a primitive.

Freud and many of his followers were convinced that there are definite similarities to be found between the mentality of the small child and that of the primitive. They also believed that the mind of the child operates on principles other than those which govern normal adult behavior. The theory of Lévy-Bruhl, which stated an equally profound difference between the primitive and the modern civilized mentality, seemed to furnish a clear proof of the psychoanalytic conceptions. Further similarities were discovered between the mental operations of the schizophrenic mind and those of children and primitives. This mental disease was said to be characterized by " archaic" and "magic" ways of thinking and thus to be the manifestation of a "regression" to a much lower level of mentality than is that of the sane person.

This theory rests in fact, on a rather weak foundation. As I have tried to explain elsewhere, it is possible only if the whole system of psychoanalytic psychology is admitted as true. The psychoanalytic school has never considered the possibility that the observations referred to, which are correct to some extent, might allow for a different explanation.

Such an explanation could be found by considering that like responses are bound to ensue when the human mind encounters like situations. It is not difficult to realize that the primitive and the child find themselves insofar in very similar situations as they are both faced with an unknown, mysterious, and threatening reality. The schizophrenic, too, finds himself in a new world with which he is almost as little acquainted as the child with his world.

A short time ago one of the pillars on which this psychoanalytic conception rests has been pulled down. Lévy-Bruhl had already modified his theory notably in many of his later works. After his death appeared an article which published some of the notes this scholar had made in preparation of a new book which he was never to write.[3] This posthumous publication amounts to a thorough recantation.

One cannot but admire the intellectual honesty with which the octogenarian scholar intended to admit the error to which he had fallen prey. There is, he declares, no such thing as a primitive or archaic logic.

---

3 "Les carnets de L. Lévy-Bruhl," *Revue Philosophique,* LXXII (1947) 258. For a more detailed discussion of the implications for psychology and psychiatry, cf. R. Allers, "Über die Begriffe eines 'archaischen Denkens' und 'der Regression,'" *Wiener Zschr.f.Nervenheilhunde u. deren Grezgebiete,* I (1948) 309.

The primitive mind operates according to the same principles which we know. The law of participation does not exist. He had made the mistake, Lévy-Bruhl says, "to make the facts speak, instead of letting them speak by themselves." This is tantamount to saying that he had been blinded by certain preconceived ideas the truth of which he took so much for granted that he neglected to examine their trustworthiness.

The argument which the theory of Lévy-Bruhl seemed to furnish has thus come to naught. This will not convince those who have availed themselves of this argument; they welcomed the statements of Lévy-Bruhl because they fitted with their already firmly established convictions, and these are so deeply rooted that they will withstand even greater shocks. They are rooted, in fact, not in empirical evidence but in preconceived philosophies.

The argument that human nature or, at least, human ways are so different that one cannot truly understand the mentality of a foreign people, particularly if the language, too, is widely different, is not of a kind to carry much weight. Those who tell us that we do not understand what the other peoples think or feel are at pains to prove this contention by explaining carefully what it is the others mean and we do not understand. But this seems to show that we are capable of understanding, if we only apply ourselves to this task and do not rashly read into the statements of the foreigners our own meanings.[4]

The approach to such problems has been vitiated by the preponderant "subjectivism." By this I refer to the habit of considering, almost exclusively in psychological and anthropological analysis, the way the mind is supposed to function without regard to the contents with which this mind is preoccupied. In other words: the differences one observes in human conduct may as well spring from differences in mental operations as from differences of the world in which individuals or peoples exist.

For a man to be fearful when he lives in a world of relatively great security is, probably, a symptom of his somehow abnormal mentality; but to be fearful if one is actually surrounded by a number of dangers, especially without the possibility of either foreseeing them or of warding them off effectively, is not a "symptom" but a perfectly normal form of behavior. In such cases we do, indeed, take account of the environmental circumstances. But the same consideration applies in numerous

4 See, for instance, S. Hayakawa, *Language in Action* (New York, 1939).

other cases in which such a consideration is usually disregarded. If one were, for instance, to ask oneself whether he would not behave much as the primitive does, were one to live under the same conditions, with the same lack of knowledge and the same deficiency of technological means, one might easily discover that the apparently unintelligible behavior and the curious utterances of the primitive would then be his own. There is nothing strange in man's hitting on magical explanations and magical procedures if he is surrounded by mysterious forces the action of which he can neither calculate nor turn to his advantage.

Perhaps the best illustration of this subjectivism in psychology is furnished by certain classifications of psychological or personality types. Most of these typologies may be characterized as being "formal," insofar as they are based on the preponderance of certain mental functions or general attitudes. But a person is not at all characterized by his being labelled, say, as an introvert. There are many differences among the so called introverts. And these differences depend on that particular aspect of reality, inner reality be it, with which the person is primarily concerned.[5]

A consideration of the facts as they are and not as they appear in the light of some preconceived philosophies may, therefore, make us confident that human nature is everywhere and at all times the same. If it can be shown that the demands of a moral code are at all "commensurate" to human nature, then they must stay so under all circumstances.

We might even go one step farther. It might be possible to develop from an analysis of human nature a series of moral demands with which man has to comply to be wholly himself, that is, to achieve the highest degree of perfection of which he is capable.[6] Such attempts have been made, in fact, recently, on the part of a philosopher and on that of psychologists or psychiatrists. Paul Weiss has not yet stated his ethical conceptions; but the work which he intends as a sort of prolegomena to such an ethics is sufficiently indicative of his viewpoint. Apart from the general metaphysics on which this conception is based, it may be briefly characterized as aiming at the establishment

5 A "material" typology has been established by E. Spranger and modified as well as been made practical by G. W. Allport, in his *Personality* (New York, 1937).

6 Perfection means here the greatest possible degree of actualization, and thus does not refer only to moral perfection.

of an universally valid, system of morals developed from, an analysis of human nature.[7]

Erich Fromm is more explicit. It is not necessary to discuss here his special ideas and his criticism of what he terms "authoritarian ethics." It suffices to point out that he, too, is dissatisfied by and worrying about the hopeless relativism in which modern ethics has become involved. His ethics is strictly naturalistic. But it differs from other such proposals by its claim of universal validity. This validity is to be ensured by founding ethics on the study of human nature and deriving therefrom a system of rules which man ought to obey if he is to attain his perfection and the best possible state of society.[8]

It is interesting to note that even a man so completely addicted to the tenets of Freudian psychoanalysis, as Dr. E. Bergler is, arrives at similar conclusions, at least on one point. He defends monogamy and, to a certain extent, the lastingness, though not, of course, the indissolubility, of marriage. It does not matter that he bases his argument on the "Oedipus complex" which he believes to be a common and inevitable factor in human life. The point is that he, too, believes in a moral precept as deducible from an analysis of human nature.[9]

If such an analysis were to proceed without any naturalistic or other prejudices, it might furnish useful results. One would have to renounce any foregone conclusions and start with a descriptive study. This requires a good deal of self criticism as well as that one free oneself from the current ideas of psychology and anthropology. Whatever its difficulties, the task is important. That it has been considered sufficiently by moral philosophy is doubtful.

Among other things, it is highly to be desired that psychology be more occupied with the study of volitional performances than it is today. The work done in this field is mostly vitiated by a marked preference for the "approach from below." This approach is chosen not so much because it is believed to be "scientific," although this idol plays a great role,[10] but chiefly because of the underlying philosophy which denies free will even before it has come to ascertain the facts.

7 P. Weiss, *Nature and Man* (New York, 1947).

8 E. Fromm, *Man for Himself* (New York, 1947).

9 E. Bergler, *Divorce Won't Help* (New York, 1948).

10 R. Allers, "Ideas, Ideals, and Idols," *Conflicts of Power in Modern Culture*, ed. L. Bryson, L. Finkelstein, and R. McIver (New York, 1947) p. 475.

Our understanding of volitional operations is not furthered by renaming them results of "conditioning." The psychologists have, generally, a much too high opinion of the explanatory value of the notion of "conditioned reflexes" which as have shown, for instance, E. Straus[11] and K. Goldstein[12] are in truth rather different from what psychologists believe them to be. Like many other ideas cherished by the psychologists, this one, too, belongs to the neurophysiological mythology which, unfortunately, holds so large a place in modern psychological thought.

If the statements on motivation and volition are not couched in the language of such a more or less fantastic "brain-mythology," they are dependent on the psychoanalytic conceptions of the instincts and their transformations. The use of the terms must not, but usually does, mean also an adoption of the ways of thought. Psychoanalysis, as conceived of by Freud and his school, is unavoidably deterministic. It also considers conscious motivations as misleading and as not representing the forces which in fact prompt human behavior. Because of this and other features, the approach to a "moral psychology" is closed to this manner of looking at the human mind.

The emphasis either on neural processes or on instincts reveals the influence philosophical convictions exercise on the formation of psychological ideas. The differences between the various schools of psychology are fundamentally differences of the underlying philosophies. The categories by the means of which observations are stated are not imposed on the student by the facts; they are derived from philosophical prejudices.

All this is, however, not tantamount to a denial of the usefulness of the work done by the psychologists. Our knowledge of habit formation, for instance, of attitudes, of the influence of emotional states, especially of such one might call "chronic," has been notably broadened, and it would be a serious neglect if moral philosophy would fail to take account of these things. But it is also evident that many problems are still awaiting adequate study, although they are of primary importance for our understanding of moral behavior. There is almost nothing to be found on the psychological factors at work in the building up of virtues or, for that matter, the psychology of vices either.

11 E. Straus, *Die Einheit der Sinne* (Berlin, 1932).

12 K. Goldstein, *The Organism* (New York, 1938); *Human Nature in the Light of Psychopathology* (Cambridge, Mass., 1939).

If one turns from psychology, as the individual aspect of anthropology, to cultural anthropology, one does well to realize that the advance of these studies is owed not so much to the, indeed great, widening of factual knowledge as to the improvement of methods of inquiry.

The cultural anthropologist has leaned to view a culture, as it were, "from within" and has come to realize that such a phenomenon cannot be understood unless it be considered in its totality.

The procedure used by almost all students of these matter previously consisted mainly in viewing one or the other side of a culture without integrating it with all the others. Furthermore, they often evaluated such civilizations simply by comparing them with their own, which resulted in labelling the former "inferior." By viewing a culture "from within" one discovers that many traits which appear, at first sight, either shocking or unintelligible have their definite place and significance within the totality of such a culture.

This approach has deepened markedly our understanding of foreign peoples. It has not, however, proceeded far enough or become sufficiently general for most people to realize that the same approach must be used also in regard to varieties of our own civilization, that is, that the type of western civilization represented, for instance, by France or by Spain, has to be understood on its own terms, in the light of the history, the folkways, the general attitude of the population.

Feeling that they had failed to do justice to foreign civilizations, the cultural anthropologists have become anxious to avoid what they call "ethnocentrism."[13] By this term one refers to the natural inclination to judge of other civilizations by making one's own the measure, automatically assuming that it is also simply the best. There is no doubt that such an attitude may become and has become an obstacle to understanding. But this fact does not allow us to conclude that, therefore, all civilizations are of the same value. It may happen that one's preference for his own civilization is objectively correct, although its statement rests on a purely subjective factor. Subjectivity and objectivity are not simply correlated to falsehood and truth. A man may hit on the truth also when arguing from false premises. The mere fact of preference has no direct relation to the goodness of the thing preferred. It is a logical error to assume that a thing cannot be better than another

13 See, for instance, M. Herskovits, *Man and His Works* (New York, 1948), pp. 68 ff. and passim.

only because I happen to like it. But this is precisely the way in which many cultural anthropologists seem to reason.

This confusion is rather amazing. One should expect that ever so little ability in handling the rules of logic would help to avoid falling prey to this fallacy. So, one reads not without astonishment:

It is not chance that a philosophy of cultural relativism . . . has had to wait the development of adequate ethnographic knowledge. As long as the customs of peoples could not be studied in terms of their context of values, they of necessity had to be evaluated in terms of the ethnocentrism of the appraiser.[14]

The latter part of the passage is, indeed, correct. But the first is open to serious objections. Particularly, it is not true that the development of ethnographic knowledge led to cultural relativism. Rather, this view is but the application of the generally prevailing relativism to the special field of ethnographic knowledge. In other words, the fact that different peoples conceive in different manners of the order of value has nothing to do with the question whether or not there is an objectively justified order of values. It must be admitted previously that no such order exists, or, at least is discoverable, for such a conclusion to be drawn.

The defenders of "cultural relativism" deceive themselves when the believe that their work furnishes a confirmation of even a foundation to this relativism. It does this only if its results are interpreted in terms of such a relativism. The argument is a classical example of circular reasoning.

From the eminently valuable data collected by the incessant and self sacrificing work of the cultural anthropologists conclusions may be drawn which differ strangely from those these authors themselves present. It seems rather that the material of ethnography supplies quite an amount of evidence in favor of the thesis that there is a common stock of values found everywhere. The differences in moral evaluations are not so much such of content as of extent.

This may be illustrated, for instance, by considering "love of one's neighbor."

To love his neighbor man was enjoined not only in the Old Covenant If the commandment received its full significance only by the teachings of Christ, to extend love even to one's enemies, it has been somehow written into the hearts of men at all times. The change in the

14 *Ibid.* p. 78.

advance of mankind is not the birth of the idea that one has to love one's neighbor, but the growing width of the definition.

For the primitive, the neighbor is only a member of his own tribe. Later, he may be of other tribes with whom the former is on friendly terms. The stranger, the guest, the tradesman are gradually included. With the spreading of the Roman Republic first, then the Empire, the notion is still more widened. Many inhabitants of the countries outside of Italy become Roman citizens; St. Paul is an example. Afterwards, every subject of the Empire is considered *civis Romamus*. The Stoa develops the idea of humanity and of human dignity inherent in man as such, independently of nation or social status.

The notion of a certain obligation of man in regard to some of his fellows is found everywhere. Finally, with Christianity, even the kind of relations between man and man, whether of friendship or of enmity, cease to be relevant.

The development of other moral notions runs parallel to that of the neighbor. There is, probably, no civilization however primitive which would not forbid murder. But murder may be defined in a wider and a narrower sense. To kill a slave is not deemed murder; he is the property of the master and not recognized as being endowed with rights. Nor is it thought murder to kill the member of a hostile tribe but a meritorious act of "preventive war," so to speak. There may be other factors. The primitive warrior has a definite esteem for the prowess of his actual or potential enemy; thus he enhances his greatness by killing the other. He may do more, and proceed to feed on his enemy. Anthropology has shocked all who come across it. But one has to consider that this custom is not a failure to recognize the other's worth; quite to the contrary, in the anthropophagic feast those who participate believe that they will acquire something of the valor of the dead. Paradoxical though it seems, one might risk the statement that the anthropophage manifests a greater appreciation of human worth than does the slaveholder.

A moral idea may be recognized but expressed in a manner which is so alien to the observer that he does not identify the idea. It would be an interesting topic to discuss how charity manifested itself at different times and under varying con ditions. It is questionable whether a member of the early Church would recognize charity in the forms in which it appears today.

If one starts with the presumption that differences of civilization bring about, necessarily, differences in basic evaluations, and if he thus makes evaluation totally dependent on culture, one may overlook the fundamental identity of the recognized moral values because of the far going differences in their applications or manifestations.

Could it be ascertained that the basic values are everywhere and at all times the same, a severe blow could be dealt to the conception that all morality is but a product of the prevailing social and cultural conditions. That this is not the case is shown by the fact of differences existing within one and the same civilization. The existence, side by side, of widely different ideas on morality during the first centuries of the Christian era might be used for an illustration.

It is obvious that the material situations which demand the application of certain basic principles may vary considerably. New obligations may arise because new situations emerge. One need only remember that in times of war forms of behavior become obligatory which in peacetime are almost non existent. Thus, suspiciousness, attention to what another says, those with whom he has contacts, denunciation, secrecy, attain an importance which they do not possess outside of such unusual conditions and some things may become duties which in normal times have to be avoided.

Certain social and political conditions create new duties and make their fulfillment imperative. Thus, we have the obligation for dynastic loyalty in monarchies, or that of intelligent political cooperation in democracies.

Several of the remarks made above pertain to what had been called the "apologetic" approach. This approach has also been characterized as a negative one. It is negative because its emphasis is on the refutation of the claims made by the other side, and it carries conviction much more with those of one's own side than with the opponents.

Important though this approach is, it has its definite drawbacks. It is, so to speak, secondary; that is, it is a reply and therefore dependent on the attack. It seldom forestalls attacks, since this can be done, indeed, only by a more positive procedure. One has to prove the legitimacy of one's position with sufficient reliable evidence so as to render it impregnable, so far as this is feasible. The apologetic reply creates, almost inevitably, the impression that it is forced on the defender by the attack and is, as it were, something of an afterthought.

The sharpest criticism of traditional morals comes from those who profess a psychologistic interpretation of moral behavior. In recent times, this view has chiefly operated by means of the "genetic approach."

It should be noted that this theory does not necessarily lead to ethical relativism, though there is generally a close association of the two notions. It has been reported above that there are today some who conceive of founding a non relativistic system of ethics on inquiries of such a nature.

The genetic approach is held today in the highest esteem. The theory of evolution on one hand, the ideas of Freud on the other have contributed to the common belief that genetic analysis is all that can and ought to be done.

However, it is well to bear in mind that, as J. Laird remarked,[15] a genetic argument is on nothing but on genesis.

And the late Morris Cohen emphasized that no however detailed genetic analysis can dispense us from a careful study and description of the state whose origin we thus explain.[16]

In view of the fact that most of the "psychological critique" of traditional ethics uses arguments based on genetic analysis and theories derived therefrom, a brief consideration of the "genetic approach" and its relevance is not out of place.

By heeding such remarks as mentioned in the foregoing paragraph one is rendered aware of a serious gap in knowledge which cannot fail to exist if the genetic approach is the only one used. If we know, as evolutionists, all factors and antecedents of the cat, we still do not know the cat. By being told all about the instinctual forces entering into a work of art or a poem, we learn nothing of its essence. No inquiry into the psychogenesis of a sentiment of guilt can make us realize what it means to feel guilty. The most detailed discussion of the social and psychological conditions back of the phenomenon of conscience leaves us in the dark concerning its nature. To identify conscience with the performances of a hypothetical "super ego" may be interesting, perhaps give us some insight, but it does not help us truly to understand what conscience is.

---

15 Laird, *Problems of the Self* (London, 1917).

16 M. R. Cohen, *Studies in Philosophy and Science* (New York, 1949).

It is particularly the almost general acceptance of Freudian views which has, more than anything else, brought about the preference for the genetic approach. The particular conception of genesis in Freudian doctrine deserves brief consideration because a certain methodological fallacy becomes more apparent here than in other instances.

The procedure of genetic analysis, as employed by Freud and his school, rests on the assumption that the discovery of significance is also that of causes. Analysis is supposed to trace back any phenomenon of the mind or of human behavior to certain early antecedents which are said to be expressed or "symbolized" by the phenomenon analyzed. Thus, part of a dream is said to symbolize some infantile experience and, at the same time, to be caused by it. It is, of course, true that this particular phenomenon would not have emerged, if it is a "symbol," had the antecedent experience not taken place. But this is not the same thing as to say that this previous occurrence is the cause of the fact under consideration.

It seems to me that back of such statements is a confusion in the notion of causation. The antecedent symbolized is the material cause of the so called symbol. But it need not be the efficient cause. That which is expressed need not be the reason why expression is sought.

The same criticism applies to the reasonings of certain students of cultural anthropology. It deserves to be noted in passing that, the opposition of eminent scholars, notwithstanding, there is a close alliance of psychoanalysis and cultural anthropology.[17] This is, it seems, more than a coincidence or the effect of personal idiosyncrasies. It is indicative of a deep-seated likeness, in the mode of thinking here and there.

If human behavior and human work, all that could be comprised under the Hegelian term of the "objective spirit," are envisaged exclusively as "expressions," that is, if absolute preference is given to the "subjectivistic" angle, the consequence cannot be but a thoroughgoing relativism.

The claim that the moral code must change with changing cultural conditions is the most evident manifestation of this relativism.

A few years ago Dr. Chisholm stated this idea in a rather blunt manner. His argument may be summarized by saying that he starts

17 Cf. e.g. C. Kluckhohn, "Some Aspects of Navaho Infancy and Early Childhood," *Psychoanalysis and the Social Sciences*, ed. G. Róheim (New York, 1947) 37.; *Personality in Nature, Society and Culture*, ed. C. Kluckhohn (New York, 1948).

from the premise that mental health must be preserved. Secondly, that mental health is endangered by conflicts which the individual proves unable to solve. Conflicts are found in the history of most persons afflicted with mental troubles, especially of the kind termed neurotic. Conflict, therefore, ought to be eliminated as far as possible. It arises chiefly between the "natural inclinations" of man and the demands made on him by the existing moral code. Since the natural inclinations cannot be changed, the moral code must be changed according to man's needs.[18]

In this reasoning there is an obvious fallacy. It is based on the cases the psychiatrist or the social worker or the psychologist in a child guidance clinic observes. It is true that many of these cases have suffered and do suffer from all sorts of conflicts and that these apparently are important factors in the genesis and the continuation of their symptoms. It is equally true that among "problem children," maladjusted older people, delinquents, and other such types, there are many who show a history of "frustration." But there are much more people who are involved in conflicts or have been exposed to frustration and are neither notably neurotic nor maladjusted. These people, however, are unknown to the observers. Hence, it follows that the conclusions drawn with so much assurance rest on a rather unreliable basis.

In surveying these discussions one is struck by a curious inconsistency on the part of the critics of the traditional morality. They are, largely, the same men who argue, and not without violence, against the notion of a stable and unchanging human nature. Progress, as they understand it, is not only an increase of scientific and technological knowledge, but a gradual change of human nature for the better. Thinly disguised, the old notion of an "infinite perfectibility" of man, as advocated by Condorcet, is easily recognized. But, suppose that human nature had changed – which in fact it has not – so as to find difficult the obedience to the moral code, it still does not follow that this code is false. One might as well conclude that man has to change further, so as to become again capable of making the moral precepts the rules of his conduct.

If this argument does not occur to the prophets of a new morality, it is because they envision progress as a rectilinear movement and as a prolongation, so to speak, of evolution into history. The similarity

18 G. Chisholm, "The Psychiatry of Enduring Peace and Social Progress (The Reestablishment of Peacetime Society,)" *Psychiatry*, IX (1946).

of this idea with those of Freudian psychology, as outlined above, is striking. In the case of this sort of theory in cultural anthropology one observes the same identification of evolution and history as in Freud.

Not all "naturalistic" minded scholars, however, indulge in this way of thinking. One of the outstanding naturalists of our times, Prof. Julian Huxley, writes: "Progress is a major fact of past evolution; but it is limited to a few selected stocks. It may continue in the future, but it is not inevitable; man, by now become the trustee of evolution, must work and plan if he is to achieve further progress for himself and so for life."[19] Although this reads at first as if the author would, too, envisage "progress," that is, history as a "prolongation" of organic evolution, one has but to ponder a little on his words to discover that this is not so. Evolution has never, nor could it, required the conscious and intentional cooperation of the evolving species. In these words, there is not only the recognition of a definitely new mode of "progress," as set over against the "origin of species," but also of the unique place man holds in the order of nature.

There are other inconsistencies too. The inclinations the frustration of which is considered as so harmful, are selected according to some principle difficult to discover and more difficult to justify. If some person's inclination for committing theft is frustrated, nobody thinks it wrong. Also, aggressiveness is viewed as a secondary result of frustration, though in older times it was believed to belong to the basic equipment of human nature. After the legend of the "noble savage" lost credit, it became the fashion to imagine primitive man, the cave dweller, as a brutal, cruel, highly aggressive being. One cannot see, indeed, why one inclination should be considered as more "natural" than another. Little perspicacity is necessary to realize that the so called frustrations of modem man refer mostly to sexual behavior. The reform of morals which is urged, is mostly one of sexual behavior. One critic of the famous "Kinsey Report" has emphatically pointed out: if a similar report were made on, e.g., the frequency of theft, nobody would think of drawing the consequences many have found fit to draw from Dr. Kinsey's data.

Back of all these ideas is the ethical relativism which prevails today. This relativism is, of course, not a product of modern cultural anthropology, as some seem to believe, but a characteristic of a mentality which developed since the beginning of the modern age, or rather

19 J. Huxley, *Evolution, A Modern Synthesis* (New York, 1942) p. 578,

preceded it. The discovery of the great differences of moral codes in various places, added to the older knowledge of such differences in history, was only a corroboration of and an argument for the relativistic conception.

The history of ethical relativism has yet to be written. Those who adhere to this view have pointed out that late medieval nominalism is one of the ancestors of relativism. In doing so, they distort usually the meaning of these medieval systems. It is, however, true that nominalism has prepared the terrain. The story is indubitably much more complicated. Both the idealistic trend and the reaction against it, in the shape of positivism and pragmatism, have contributed in bringing forth the relativistic position.

It had not been the intention of idealism to undermine the certitude of moral precepts. But in denying to any endeavor surpassing the boundaries of reason the right to claim "scientific" certitude, Kant seriously endangered the convincingness of any attempt to establish an objectively true system of morality.

Another factor in the development of modern relativism is the idea of "progress." Its influence goes much farther than is generally acknowledged. The view that the latest stage is also the highest hitherto attained, and by the fact of being the latest proves itself to be better than any of its precedents, has done much to make the theory of evolution popular.[20] Succession becomes evolution, that is, progress. We are said to possess today a civilization superior to all which went before. Here is the link between the ideas of progress and ethnocentrism. That the latter had to be abandoned, as a methodological fallacy, has not been seen as a warning against the former or, at least, its uncritical generalizations.

To the insufficiently clarified philosophies back of the criticism of morals is added the incapacity of the modern mind to form an ad-

20 In a novel by Th. Fontane, a once widely read German writer, an old gentleman makes more or less this remark: "I recall well when this affair with the monkeys started. That was quite something. As long as people were told that they were children of God, it did not impress them particularly. But when they heard that their grandfather had been an ape, then you ought to have seen them, how enthusiastic they waxed." The eminent sociologist and economist Werner Sombart, in commenting on this reaction, suggests that the theory of evolution was so much welcomed because it offered a splendid excuse for man's baser instincts to become alone "natural." W. Sombart (*Der Mensch*, Berlin, 1936).

equate notion of human nature. Naturalism, when dealing with man, is the most unnatural philosophy conceivable.

In no other period of human knowledge has man ever become more problematic to himself as in our own days. We have a scientific, a philosophical and a theological anthropology which know nothing of each other. The ever growing multiplicity of the particular sciences engaged n the study of man has much more confused and obscured than elucidated our concept of man.[21]

Science has failed to do what it seemed to promise, namely to furnish a frame of reference for all the various aspects of man and his existence. Relativistic, naturalistic, pragmatistic philosophies have, not been able to provide for the much desired integration.

The believers in traditional morality, in a universal natural law,[22] in one word, those who hold true the *philosophia perennis,* are the only ones who may point the way out of the present confusion. But to do so and thus to answer the call of the times, it is of imperative necessity that the reply to the criticisms brought forth by either psychology or cultural anthropology be based on independent factual research, research carried on without any particular "apologetic" intentions and without a slavish imitation of the methodologies in use. These latter are too much pervaded by the philosophical ideas back of them and latent, but influential, in the minds of so many scholars, as to allow for uncritical adoption. It is not so much the mere collection of facts, important though it be, but their interpretation and integration which counts.

Strictly methodological analysis has fallen into discredit. It is considered sterile. Only facts are valuable. But in this, very common, idea it is overlooked that the so called facts seldom are merely that, as has been stated above. To. discover the specific "coloring" by preconceived ideas, the analysis of methodology is indispensable: One need only think of the use of psychoanalytic categories in cultural anthropology to become aware of this need.

Ethics, because of its essential "in betweenness," requires reliable and extensive factual knowledge. We still have no treatise which might

21 M. Scheler, *Die Stellung des Menschen im Kosmos* (Darmstadt, 1928), pp. 13 ff. E. Cassirer, could repeat these words in 1944 as still describing the situation, *An Essay on Man* (New Haven, 1944).

22 For an interesting restatement of the idea of natural law, see M. Hillenbrand, *Power and Morals* (New York, 1949).

achieve for our times what the *tractatus de homine* of St. Thomas did for the past.

The emergence and the success of the, conceptions usually subsumed under the title of "existentialism" – although these ideas differ so much that to put them together is a rather questionable enterprise – are a proof of the general need for a new philosophy of human nature. To a large part, however, these existentialistic philosophies are unable to comply with the demands of the times. They are reactions, indeed, but at the same time, very much children of their age, subjectivistic, relativistic, atheistic.

A comprehensive, truly philosophical anthropology which would also render account of the facts – *salvare apparentia* – still a desideratum. Without such a foundation, the science of ethics cannot either cope with. the present situation or successfully answer its critics.

Man needs to understand himself again. He must be given back the assurance of his personal worth. Without knowing of this worth he cannot withstand the "slings and arrows of outrageous fortune." Without consciousness of his unique dignity he cannot be expected to overcome manifold temptations. To act according to the principles of ethics he must believe that he is capable of such achievement. But he will not conceive of himself in such a manner, as long as he thinks of himself only as "a little above the white rat" and not, as he well might, as "a little below the angels."

THE DIALECTICS OF FREEDOM

The formula, "freedom and authority," suggests, as do many such formulas of similar structure, that there exists between the two terms a perfect opposition and that they are mutually exclusive. They may be, indeed, defined in such a manner as to make this opposition appear inevitable. But it is not certain that they must be thus defined.

Nor is it certain that to an opposition of terms must correspond in reality the same opposition of the referents. It is submitted in this essay that this mutual exclusiveness does not exist, and that, to the contrary, the two terms are correlated to each other so as to make each of them, or rather each of the referents, dependent on the other. A relation entailing interdependence and contradiction is called dialectical. Hence, the title.

The thesis, then, is that freedom, to be truly what the name means, requires the existence of authority and even brings it forth. Likewise, that authority is meaningless unless exercised over free persons.

THE PHILOSOPHICAL STANDPOINT

How such a problem as that of "freedom and authority" appears to the individual student depends on his general philosophical standpoint. Terms are equivocal; ideas allow for very different interpretations. Each author takes for granted his own interpretation and his own terminology, and assumes tacitly that every other one uses terms in the same sense. I shall, therefore, define as far as possible the fundamental standpoint from which the problem will here be envisaged.

As it is impossible to give a detailed explanation, let alone a formal justification of these fundamental ideas, I shall simply list a number of propositions in dogmatic form. This procedure will, or so I hope, have at least the advantage of rendering impossible arguments arising because of equivocations.

The following propositions, then, are fundamental for the argument of this essay:

1. It pertains to man's nature that he have a free will. If this is not assumed, all discussions on freedom or similar problems become meaningless. If he is not free, man is caught in the inexorable cosmic

process, and it may as well be his fate to be made the passive subject of totalitarian power as to indulge in the illusion of liberty.

2. Man's will exercises a "ruling power" – *dominium politicum*, says Aquinas – over all appetitions. If man is in full possession of his capacities, he need never become the passive playball of some forces, not even of his "instincts," the existence of which in the normal adult is anyhow questionable.

3. Like all appetition, will aims at the realization of the good. By virtue of the fact that it still is to be realized, the good which is the end pursued by will is not yet real. All will aims at a future state of affairs, which is judged "better" than that existing at present. But no judgment can have a compulsory power over will which, while still aiming at the realization of some good, is not forced to aim at that good which is judged as greater: *Video meliora proboque, deteriora sequor*.

4. Among the goods which are possible ends of will there are some whose goodness consists in nothing other than their ability to provide satisfaction. Their goodness depends largely, though, perhaps, not exclusively, on their relation to man's desires. There are others which "exist" – in the peculiar mode in which values and other non material things may be said to exist[1] – independently of their ability to provide satisfaction. They are good because they embody "objective values."

5. The objective values form a definite order which originates from the intrinsic nature of the values. This order is, however imperfectly, discoverable. The theory of "relativism" in regard to values is unfounded, not countenanced by facts, and deleterious to any attempt at defending any view on human affairs as being better than another. Especially, if there is no objective order of values, does it become impossible to maintain that man is entitled to liberty or that a liberal political constitution offers any advantages over one which turns man into a mere atom of a greater whole. Without the acceptance of the idea of an objective axiological order, criticism of ideas not approved by ourselves becomes utterly meaningless. We then have no answer to the contention that others may prefer what appears as execrable to ourselves.

For the end of the present discussion it does not make any difference in what manner the objective order is conceived. I am convinced, personally, that axiological objectivism requires the idea of a *summum bonum*. But as long as it is admitted that some sort of objective order

1 Cf. Nicolai Hartmann, *Das Problem des geistigen Seins*, Walter de Gruyter, Berlin, 2nd edition, 1949.

of values exists and may be, however faintly, envisaged, a discussion on what is better and what worse will make sense.

THREE ASPECTS OF FREEDOM

A well known distinction opposes "freedom from" to "freedom for." The former term refers to the absence of all obstacles rendering impossible or insufficient the satisfaction of the so called "basic needs." If one is agreed on these needs, the types of freedom for may be determined. The notion, however, entails at least two difficulties.

The first becomes visible when one considers that every freedom for may encounter obstacles. Freedom for presupposes, therefore, a peculiar kind of freedom from. Obstacles which oppose the satisfaction of basic needs appear as simple denials of the corresponding freedom from. This freedom is itself basic and not related secondarily to another freedom. But what is comprised under the heading of freedom for, that is, for ends not related to basic needs, requires as a condition that there be a secondary freedom, secondary in the sense that it is subservient to the other. In other words, the distinction is not of that clarity which some seem to attribute to it.

The second difficulty is more serious. Satisfaction of basic needs is not definable because of the wide range from the lowest degree of satisfaction to any higher degree. One has only to consider the meaning of "freedom from want." It is impossible to indicate how far supply must be increased to fulfil the condition of freedom from want. There is the level of mere subsistence on which the basic needs for food, shelter, and so forth, are indubitably satisfied. But an existence on the mere subsistence level is not at all "satisfactory."

Any freedom may be viewed, first, as determined by the ends for the realization of which man is made free; and, secondly, in regard to the degree in which such realization is possible. The first consideration may be called "vectorial," the second "scalar." Most discussions on freedom take account only of the vectorial aspect; they seem to presuppose that freedom is essentially unlimited. From the remarks made by several writers on these problems, one gathers that they apparently view any restriction of freedom as unjustified, and fear that even a slight restriction threatens freedom. But limitation is not only not tantamount to derogating freedom, but is a condition without which freedom cannot exist.

Apart from the twofold aspect of being determined by its vectors and its scalars, there is a third aspect of freedom which often seems to be neglected. The possession of freedom on the part of the individual and its recognition on the part of the community or the legal constitution is one thing; the exercise of freedom another.

In ordinary life man recognizes that there may be conditions under which fall use of his freedoms is either unadvisable or wrong. The general freedom or right to say what one thinks, may be, and often is, restricted by the demands of prudence and of charity, not to mention custom. Freedom is not threatened nor abrogated, if account is taken of such conditions. In fact, nobody but some extremist will claim that his freedom is curtailed by such considerations. Neither does man, generally, admit that he or any of his fellows is free to do evil. It is tacitly understood that freedom is only for good.

One has, therefore, to distinguish a subjective and formal side of freedom, on one hand, and a material and objective, on the other. Subjectively and formally, man may be free to titter any sentiment, opinion, judgment, on anything whatsoever. Materially and objectively he may be subject to restrictions, both in regard to vectors and scalars.

RELATIVISM AND CHANGING HUMAN NATURE

The recognition of limiting conditions does not contradict the principle stated above that values are objective and stand in a recognizable order. The changing conditions allowing or restricting freedom are sometimes used as an argument in favor of relativism when they appear successively in history or simultaneously in different civilizations. These facts are alleged as a proof of human nature being subject to change; man has no longer, according to this view, the same nature he had thousands of years ago, and it is hoped that his nature will change to the better the further civilization progresses.

That this change, should it take place at all, will be for the better is, of course, a mere postulate or even nothing other than a fond hope. It is part of the creed of progress as the eighteenth century imagined it. However, none of the enthusiastic advocates of progress, so numerous in the seventeenth and eighteenth centuries, believed in a changing human nature. *Les philosophes* thought rather of human nature as essentially good, of this goodness realized in a "state of nature" and deteriorated by social and cultural factors. How this good human nature could ever give birth to such deteriorating forces remains an unexplained mystery. The modern idea of progress, though a descendant of that alive around 1750, is no longer the same as it was at first; it is the product of an unholy alliance between the notion of moral and cultural perfection and that of biological evolution.

It is necessary that a few words be said on this particular interpretation of "progress." In this regard, the following quotation appears to the point:

> . . . the problem of values must be faced. Man differs from any previous dominant type in that he can consciously formulate values. And the realization of these in relation to the priority determined by whatever scale of values is adopted, must be accordingly added to the criteria of biological progress, once advance has reached the human level. Furthermore, the introduction of such criteria based upon values . . . alters the direction of progress. It might perhaps be preferable to say that it alters the level on which progress occurs.

These lines are taken from the concluding chapter in Professor Julian Huxley's work, *Evolution*.[2] Only one additional remark seems necessary. Professor Huxley justly says that the "level is altered on which progress occurs." One has, however, to consider that with a shift of level is associated also a shift of categories. That is, progress assumes a totally different character on the new level, even though it remains progress nonetheless. Aristotelian or Thomistic Scholasticism would insist, and I believe correctly, that progress is not an unequivocal but an "analogical" term.

Whatever formulation one may prefer, one thing stands out clearly: that to equate progress in civilization with evolution amounts to the logical fallacy of a *metabasis eis allo genos*.

It is because of this fallacy that the advocates of a "changing human nature" become involved in self contradiction. It is hardly an exaggeration if one attributes to these men the idea that the progress from older forms of political constitution to that of democracy entails not only a definite advance and improvement of human situations, but also a change of human nature: progress gives birth to the "democratic man."

---

2 'Julian Huxley, *Evolution*, Harper & Brothers, New York London, 1942, p. 575.

But were human nature to change, it could not do so in a sudden cataclysm. Man would change gradually and some individuals would change more and others less. Some parts of mankind or even of a nation would advance more quickly than others. The effect must be a growing inequality. The final result might well be the emergence of a race of "supermen," rather as Nietzsche conceived of these fantastic creatures. Men would have to cease to believe that they are "born equal," or each of the new race will have to arrogate the name of *homo sapiens* to himself, while degrading his less fortunate brother to the status of *homo servus*.

Of course, nothing of this kind will happen. The talk about changing human nature is, after all, but an outcome of a certain benevolent but improvident enthusiasm which one need not take seriously, were it not that it apparently appeals to many uncritical minds.

THE COMPLEXITY OF TRUTH

It is the uncritical mind to which many things are "self evident." It would be well if both the philosopher and the average person realized that their most cherished beliefs may not be as well founded as they love to think. What is evident to an orthodox follower of Lenin fails to convince a Western democrat. The latter's conviction that "men are born equal" was inconceivable for a member of the privileged estates of the *ancien régime*. And not because of presumptuousness, or lust for power, or any such reasons; these men simply "knew" for sure that inequality is the law of human nature. All problems present different aspects according to the frame of reference within which they are envisaged.

It is not otherwise with the conception of freedom. If one distinguishes with Mr. T. G. Weldon[3] three fundamentally different conceptions of the State – the Democratic, the Organic, and the Power State – the consequences differ considerably in regard to the interpretation of freedom.

It is important that one see clearly in this respect. If a proposition is not of such a kind as to be truly evident – and of these there are very few; its evidence rests on that of another more general proposition which may be justly called a "prejudice" – not by way of disparagement, but in the literal sense – and it is precisely the examination of this

3 T. G. Weldon, *States and Morals*, Whittlesey House, New York, 1947.

implicit presupposition on which hinges the validity of the allegedly evident statement.

"Whatever," writes Mr. Weldon, "the authors of the Declaration of Independence asserted to the contrary, the inalienable rights of men as such to life, liberty, and the pursuit of happiness, are neither self-evident nor demonstrable."[4] Exception may be made to the last two words. It might be possible to arrive at a demonstration, if certain presuppositions are made and, perhaps, even made evident.

It may be that the authors of the Declaration of Independence were not as assertive as Mr. Weldon thinks. The American Declaration says: "We hold . . . ," but the French *Déclaration des droits de l'homme* makes a statement of unconditioned generality. One asks whether or not the authors of the Declaration were conscious of the fact that any such proposition can be held evident only within a definite frame of reference, whereas the doctrinaires of the Revolution did not hesitate to proclaim universal truth.

Theoretical discussions, as well as the handling of practical affairs, would profit were men more conscious of the primary assumptions they make, and which, once made, disappear from conscious thought because they are taken for granted.

One of the most disastrous of these implicit assumptions – though it is often not implicit at all, but openly professed, still without any further examination – is that that truth must be simple. One asks in vain, why? There is no reason whatsoever to assume that reality is essentially simple. This is so little the case that a philosopher once placed on the title page of a work the motto, *Simplex sigillum nec veri nec falsi.*[5] Simplicity has nothing to do with truth; it is not a criterion of truth, and simple statements are as much liable to be false as are complicated ones.

The problem of freedom is as complicated as any other of the fundamental questions. Its complication is of its essence) and not, as some seem to believe, the result only of recent practical situations. It is not because some people see fit to propagate Communistic ideas among the students of American schools that the problem of limitations of "freedom of speech" or "academic freedom" emerges. It has been there,

---

4 *Ibid*, p. 128.

5 J. Cohn, *Theorie der Dialektik*, F. Meiner, Leipzig, 1923.

in fact, all the time. The actual situation has only rendered more people aware of this problem.

SOME VIEWS OF FREEDOM

It seems to be the opinion of many that freedom is essentially unlimited, and that all limitations are the result of unwelcome necessities. Man in his ideal state should, according to this conception, enjoy unrestricted freedom. He could not possess unlimited scalar freedom, because the finiteness of his capacities would force him to renounce the achievement of ends he might imagine. But he would he free to move along any vector he might choose.

Such was, apparently, the idea of John Stuart Mill, He recognized, of course, that unlimited freedom is a utopian dream and that the concrete human situations render certain limitations inevitable. The inevitability of limitations, however, can be seen as founded on different reasons. Mill reveals clearly his position when he writes: "If grown persons are to be punished for not taking proper care of themselves, I would rather it were for their own sake than under the pretence of preventing them from impairing their capacity of rendering to society benefits."[6] It is not a convincing argument for an author to say that "he rather would." Mill, too, starts with some "evident truth," the nature of which is stated in the motto on the front page of his essay. It is taken from W. von Humboldt: "The great leading principle ... is the absolute and essential importance of human development in its richest diversity." Absolute and essential, indeed, only if certain presuppositions are admitted as "evident."

The intellectual climate in which Mill moved is that of an ontological nominalism, an ethical autonomism, and an anthropological subjectivism. Only within this frame of reference may Humboldt's principle be said to be absolute and essential, or may Mill feel as he does.

Mill's utilitarianism is, of course, not a primary attitude; it flows from the general philosophy indicated above. Mill's avowed preference, by virtue of which he "rather would" this and not that, cannot be derived from his utilitarian conception. It is not the utilitarian principle that allows for an answer to the question: Useful for whom?

---

6 John Stuart Mill, *On Liberty and Considerations on Representative Government,* edited by R. B. McCallum, Oxford University Press, Oxford, 1948.

Suppose that a small fraction of a large population feels quite unhappy, unless its members are permitted to preach their ideas openly and unreservedly. But the majority feels differently; most people feel unhappy when they hear these ideas preached. The conflict cannot be solved on the basis of any "felicific calculus." Nor can one appeal to "expediency," because the question, "Expedient to whom?" is unanswerable.

All such questions must be placed in a much wider frame than that of utilitarianism or, for that matter, any kind of "anthropological subjectivism." These problems require that they be envisaged from the angle of a conception within which man's place in reality can be defined.

It must be noted that this conception need not yet be metaphysics in the proper sense. The problems remain the same also when they are viewed as pertaining to a merely "phenomenal world." Man's being (*esse*) is to be (*existere*) in a world, as Heidegger justly emphasized.[7]

And it is particularly to be in association with his fellows, what Heidegger calls *Mitsein*. This is pure description. But, "to be in a world" is not yet "to face a world." Man's position is customarily viewed as if he were facing a world which would be, so to speak, "outside of himself," and of which to become or not to become a part is left to his decision. But the fact is that he is part whether or not he be aware of it. He is so much part of the world that he cannot think either of himself or of the world without taking account of the other. Man without a world is as empty as any Kantian concept without intuition, and without society he becomes undistinguishably merged with the chaos of nature[8] and never attains the actualization of his strictly human capacities and so never the "development in its richest diversity."

Consequently, there cannot exist any independence of man in regard to the laws which govern both nature and society. Whatever his freedom, it is limited by his relations to his fellows, severally and totally as society. These relations, to say it once more, are not "outside" of or added to man's nature, but constitutive of it. So also are the limitations of freedom not extraneous to freedom but essential aspects of it. Freedom exists only when and as limited.

Were freedom not limited and did its exercise not encounter resistance it would not be. The concept which considers freedom as essen-

7 M. Heidegger, *Sein und Zeit*, Niemeyer, Halle a.S., 1927, pp. 114 ff.

8 The expression is, so far as I know, Feuerbach's; the idea is, of course, much older.

tially unlimited is, in truth, the result of a "secularization" of the notion of divine freedom. But this process yields meaningless results because man has no means to understand God's freedom and in arrogating for himself what he believes to be an attribute of divine nature, he forgets that all statements of this kind are "analogical," or, as St. Augustine said, that God *melius scitur nesciendo*. By rejecting the idea of God, man does not acquire the right to credit himself with the attributes the faithful predicate of divine nature.

It is not the fact that man's nature is limited nor that many ends are mutually exclusive of each other, which bothers those who conceive of freedom as essentially unlimited. They will admit that "one cannot have the cake and eat it." Although many feel like the little boy who was asked, on his birthday, whether he wanted to listen to the band or go donkey riding, and replied: "I want to ride the donkey to the concert."

Nor are these people disconcerted too much by the fact that one cannot pursue all imaginable ends, though they believe that all opportunities should be open to all men. Goethe's advice to seek infinity by moving in all directions within finitude – *Willst Du in's Unendliche schreiten, geh' im Endlichen nach allen Seiten* – is suitable, perhaps, only for few people. What man demands is not that he become actually an infinite being, but that he be free to choose among an infinite number of ends. And choose "freely" that is, uninhibited by any conditions extraneous to his being.

But there is no infinite number of ends. However numerous, their number is finite. To the finiteness of being corresponds the finiteness of freedom, both in its vectorial and its scalar aspects.

The exercise of freedom, like that of any power in man, is possible only if there is something on which, and, therefore, against which, this exercise is effected. As Spinoza put it: *Omne ens in suo esse perseverari conatur.* The concept of a basically unlimited freedom is self-contradictory. It is not the mere fact of consideration to be taken of others and their rights which limits human freedom, as some formulas seem to imply. Thus Lord Acton wrote that freedom consists in "the assurance that every man shall be protected in doing what he believes his duty, against the influence of authorities and majorities, custom and opinion."[9] This definition will appear acceptable to many. It is, however, far from being clear and requires comment.

"Every man" can mean, obviously, only every man sound of mind and fully responsible. Neither the child nor the fool can be allowed such freedom. A schizophrenic may see his duty in doing the most unreasonable and dangerous things. He is, of course, free inasmuch as he is human; he, too, possesses "inalienable rights." But he cannot act as a responsible member of society.

It is only a part of the truth, if it is said that the fool must be prevented from doing harm so that the normal people may be protected. Obvious though this be, it is secondary. The primary thing is that the fool's actions are wrong and his sense of duty perverted.

The definition of Lord Acton, therefore, presupposes that the "sense of duty" be of the right kind, within the framework of a theory of objective right and wrong. One is led, automatically, as it were, back to the notion of the "natural law."[10]

A further qualification seems necessary. The mere "sense of duty" is not enough; it ought to read "considered sense of duty." It is easy for man to believe that he is prompted by a sense of duty, whereas, in truth, he is obeying passion or some egoistic desires. Mr. James Branch Cabell, in his *Jurgen* – a book as clever as it is fantastic – has a young man remark, "I shall always do my duty as I see it – but, then, I was born with bad eyes." Some are, maybe, born that way; but more acquire this defect later. The sense of duty or conscience must be enlightened by reason. One may dislike custom and opinion, authority and the will of majorities; but they may still voice what is just.

Without making use of some criteria outside and above one, one cannot arrive at a final judgment. If to behave as the definition of Lord Acton suggests were the essence of freedom, society would have no right whatsoever to impose restrictions on any individual, not even on the fool.[11]

9 Lord Acton, "The Theory of Freedom in Antiquity," *The History of Freedom and Other Essays*, edited by Reginald V. Lawrence and John Neville Figgis, Macmillan & Company, Ltd., London, 1907, p. 3.

10 Cf. M. J. Hillenbrand, *Power and Morals*, Columbia University Press, New York, 1949, especially pp. 69 ff.

11 A consistently subjectivistic and relativistic conception would, in fact, have no plausible reason for putting restrictions on the fool. The only reasons are those that are practical, such as protection of the others.

To discover all the implications of a "sense of duty" one would have to unravel the many threads interwoven in this idea. The influence of Christian ethics and Kantian moral philosophy, of Shaftesbury's "moral sense," and of the interpretation given to it by Hutcheson and Adam Smith, of Reid's "commonsense," and of the French Enlightenment, and others, too, would have to be appraised. For these men, moral truth appeared as not less objective than any other truth; perhaps, even more objective than many other truths. They believed in the "natural law," even if they did not stress the point.

But the notion of the "natural law" had undergone a subtle modification since the time of Thomas Hobbes. With him the natural law became a law of nature, comparable to those physics discovers. No longer is the natural law a reflex of the *lex aeterna* and implanted somehow into the minds of men, but it becomes more and more like the laws of human nature. It then depends on the view one has of nature in general and of human nature in particular, what consequences he draws. Hobbes concluded that human nature is possessed only by lust of power and fear of death; thus be arrives at his well known political philosophy. Others thought better of man's nature, and believed that his inclinations are fundamentally good; in so far as they are, they follow the "natural law," and inclination then becomes a criterion of the right. It would seem that any doctrine denying to the good some kind of objectivity must arrive at either the one or the other conception. In both cases, man's freedom is jeopardized. He becomes the slave either of a self created tyranny in the Leviathan, or of his inclinations and impulses which he has no means to evaluate. Tithe notion of an impulsive, subjective "sense of duty" be taken without qualification, it endangers the very idea of freedom. But suppose that the notion of this sense of duty be sufficiently clarified and rendered unequivocal. This sense discovers what man ought to do, what ends he ought to pursue. Therewith, however, the "autonomy" of will comes to an end. Man appears as subject to laws which are extrinsic to his nature.

This is only apparently the case. If one realizes that the opposition of ego and non ego, as it usually is made, is based on a misinterpretation of reality – of which man is part – and has to be replaced by the "dialectical" formula indicated above, the objection loses its validity. Man by obeying the law which he encounters as not his, in fact, obeys the law which is his, because he is, as a part of reality, subject to this law which governs also his own being. Not the idea of "heteronomy," to speak in Kant's terms, but that of an exaggerated "autonomy" is contrary to human nature and man's dignity.

It would seem that the best definition of freedom is still that suggested by Anselm of Canterbury: freedom is *rectitudo voluntatis propter se servata*, righteousness of will preserved for its own sake.[12] Righteousness implies that there be precepts to be observed. Freedom is significant only, if and in so far, as it is limited by principles.

The limitation is both vectorial and scalar. Reference has been made above to the obvious fact that ends may be incompatible with each other and that this incompatibility limits the exercise of freedom. Envisaged from the angle of determinant principles, this limitation appears in a new light. It is not simply a material impossibility, a result of man's restricted power, of his incapacity to pursue manifold ends at the same time, but the necessary consequence of the order of vectors. It is superficial to claim that all vectors are of the same dignity. They form an order, and thus stand to each other in the relation of higher and lower.

Utilitarianism, relativism, and similar doctrines are open to the unanswerable objection that the principle on which they rest is arbitrary and undemonstrable. Why should the "greatest happiness of the greatest number" be sought? Why should the opinion of one group, be it however numerous, prevail over that of others? Why should a man be permitted to utter publicly whatever ideas he may cherish?

AN EXAMPLE: FREEDOM OF SPEECH

To examine a special instance, some limitations of "freedom of speech" are, probably, recognized by most people. They agree, on the whole, that man is not free to slander his fellow, to use offensive language, to divulge secrets confided to him, openly to preach immorality. The idea of what constitutes improper or offensive language, or immorality, or slander, may vary. But some general agreement seems to exist.

"Freedom of speech" figures among the "inalienable rights." But what precisely this freedom implies is not defined. As the words stand, they seem to indicate that freedom of speech is an unequivocal term, hence that all speech under all conditions is covered by the formula. That this cannot be the case becomes clear, if one takes account of the recognized limitations mentioned above.

---

12 Anselm of Canterbury, *De libero arbitrio*, c. 13.

Speech, as referred to in the formula, is not the more or less pleasurable exercise of the articulatory organs. It is, first, significant utterance, and, secondly, directed at an audience. As many things may be signified, the question arises whether or not one has to do with one vector only. Is speech on this or that, to this or that person or group, one and the same thing? Its oneness becomes questionable if account is taken of what is expressed or communicated.

If freedom of speech is curtailed in some respect, it does not follow that its existence is denied or its exercise threatened. Freedom of speech does not imply that a man is free to say whatever he wishes under whatever conditions. If, therefore, it were to be claimed that certain things cannot be taught to immature minds, that other things should not be publicized, that uninhibited discussion of still other things is contrary to the interest of the community, or any such restrictive measure were taken, freedom of speech would not necessarily be endangered or abolished.

Those who are afraid of losing this freedom or of the democratic principle being imperiled, base their indignant protests on the idea that freedom of speech is a right vested in the individual person and independent of all extraneous conditions. In other words, their argument is that of an unlimited subjectivism, implying the notion of unlimited freedom. So far as restrictions are recognized, they are envisaged as imposed by necessity, not as inherent in or correlated to freedom. Obligations are enforced; they do not pertain to the nature of freedom itself.

This view is basically not too different from that of Thomas Hobbes. This philosopher, too, recognized a fundamental equality of all men, which, with him, was founded not on rights that were inherent in human nature, but on the capacity of every man to damage and kill his fellow, either by brutal force or by stealth. Mutual obligations do not arise from either human nature or a "natural law," but from dire necessity; because they are in a certain sense "unnatural," they must be imposed and maintained by the power of the tyrant.

Thomas Hobbes was not a democratic thinker. Democracy seems to imply respect for every man's person and, therefore, derives the obligation, under which everyone stands, not from necessity but from the very essence of its fundamental conception. Obligation and freedom belong together. To be obliged by the positive law, the political constitution, the moral principles, even by custom, is not in contradiction to man's freedom, and does not diminish it in the least.

It will be objected that man finds the principle of obligation in his own conscience. This is what Lord Acton implied. But conscience – like memory – is easily deceived. Many a man has deluded himself in believing that he was obeying his conscience, when in truth he was prompted by totally different motivation. If a man were to make what conscience seems to suggest at a given moment his only guide, he would make himself into the supreme lawgiver.

It is inevitable that doing one's duty be, at times, unpleasant. The "good feeling" of having done one's duty is often but a poor compensation. Nothing could be more false than the idea that men act only for the sake of some pleasure they expect as a sort of reward for having done their duty. Christian morals do not tell man to do good because he then will be rewarded; he ought to do what is good – or, in the terms of Christian doctrine, what is the will of God – simply because it is good. He is told to love his neighbor as himself, not to earn thus some reward, but because his neighbor is invested with all the dignity which is man's.

Self-interest, however "enlightened," is not a foundation of morality nor of human society. The idea of an unlimited freedom is born out of self interest, not a very enlightened one, it is true.

FREEDOM, AUTHORITY, AND DEMOCRACY

It is claimed that all restriction of freedom endangers democracy. This seems to be fallacious. True, there are forms of undemocratic political life in which freedom is restricted. But one cannot conclude therefrom, that all limitation of freedom – beyond the barest necessity – is for that reason anti democratic.

One might risk the statement that this overemphasis on freedom is the manifestation not so much of a democratic as of an adolescent mentality. No life requires more that those who lead it be mature than does democratic life. The immature mind is not fully responsible. The greater is the misfortune if the immature are entrusted with responsibility.

The essence of democracy is that – ideally speaking – every citizen be fully responsible. If democracy fails, it is because the citizens were not aware of their responsibilities. Of these responsibilities, one of the greatest is to see to it that the good be realized as far as this is within human power. As it is not an infringement of freedom to prevent a man from doing harm to himself or others, so also is it not a diminution of freedom if men are hindered from spreading evil.

Freedom is and cannot he but freedom for the good. If we are agreed that the democratic form of life is a good or that this form of life approximates the ideal form of a community more than any other, then it follows that what is contrary to this ideal is evil. And evil is to be prevented.

It is on this point that the question of authority finds its answer. Nobody doubts that some authority has to exist for the sake of maintaining civic order. The law must have its executive organs. But not all law is written. Some of the most fundamental laws are neither written nor stated explicitly. They must be observed, because they are the very laws of man himself. That he does not recognize them as such should make no difference. What is fundamental is often discovered last and through a long and laborious search.

All authority exists for the sake of an end. Authority is established that a good may be realized, or, if real, preserved. In the life of a community this good is ultimately that of all, or the common good.

Authority is the formal aspect of that power by which a person or an institution deserves to be called *auctor rei publicae*. The res publica is not simply the state or the territory or the might of a nation; it is primarily the common good. There is nothing more "public," or more in the interest of the public, than the common good.

The common good is not freedom. Freedom is, rather, that endowment of human nature which renders possible the pursuit of the good. This ought to be clear, for freedom may be as well – and has unfortunately been quite frequently – for the pursuit of evil.

Freedom is, to say it once more, not freedom for everything; it is only freedom for the good. Freedom of speech, too, falls under this definition. No college would permit any member of its faculty to give a course on "successful adultery." It does not matter whether or not this – fictitious – college professor be convinced that adultery is all to the good. That it is objectively not good, is all that counts.

It is, therefore, no deprivation of freedom if people are hindered in spreading ideas which are the opposite of what is – with cogent reasons – believed to be the good.

Who says freedom, says limitation. Who says democracy, says limitation. The limitation of which so much has been said on these pages, is something wholly other than forcefully imposed "domination" – in the sense Professor Santayana uses the term in his latest work[13] and not extrinsic to but inherent in freedom.

The very idea of democracy is perverted and deprived of its efficacy, if it is detached from its original and solid foundation on the belief in an objective order of goodness within which democracy has its definite place. If we abandon the concept of such an objective order, we lose every right to defend democracy for any reason other than that we just happen to like it.

But if such an objective order is recognized, it must be also recognized that man's freedom has its intrinsic limitations, and that freedom cannot exist unless these limitations be recognized.

One cannot have democracy and deliver it to an unbound subjectivism and relativism. Human nature is one, and so is the order of life. The "moral law within ourselves" which "aroused ever renewed admiration" in the mind of Kant, is the moral law outside of us. A man oblivious of himself and dedicated to the good, achieves by this his greatest perfection. He is free when he consents to the fact of his limited nature and realizes that obligation is not imposed from without, but is the "dialectic counterpart" of his very freedom.

Two words ought to be written so that everyone may have them before his eyes. They should adorn the walls of our schools, and they should resound in the minds of every citizen:

DEMOCRACY OBLIGES.

13 George Santayana, *Dominations and Powers*, Charles Scribner's Sons, New York, 1951.

PSYCHIATRY AND THE ROLE OF PERSONAL BELIEF

I. MENTAL HEALTH & PHILOSOPHICAL OUTLOOK

The German philosopher Johann Gottlieb Fichte first expressed an idea that one now hears quite often: "The sort of philosophy a man has depends on the sort of man he is." This is certainly true to some extent, but the reverse might also be true: The sort of man one is may depend on the sort of philosophy one has. Upon a man's philosophy depends the way in which he tries to come to terms with reality, since it is his philosophy that depicts reality to him. He sees the world and himself and, consequently, his place in and relations with the world in the light of his philosophy.[1]

Psychiatry has long known that a mental disease is not a complete novelty in the history of a person. It is not unrelated to traits, dispositions, experiences, and the effects of experiences in the person's life before the outbreak of mental disturbance. Indeed, in many cases mental disease appears to be but an increase or exaggeration of traits that were evident when the person was still normal – or at least so considered. The study of the relations between this "pre-psychotic personality," as it is called, and the type of disease to which the person falls prey is a study of great importance and one that has been very fruitful. Much of it, however, appears to be one-sided, for it considers only what might be called the formal aspects of a personality.

The same thing is true of a related, and also very important, line of inquiry, the study of psychological types. Here types may be distinguished by mental operations or prevalent tendencies. Thus the two

1 "Philosophy" as used here does not mean an elaborate system, nor does having a philosophy imply acquaintance with any of the writers on such matters. The term refers to that largely unavowed and unclarified general attitude that every person has in regard to himself, to others, and to the world in which he lives. Were the average person able to express these things, or even to figure them out for himself, the result would be his own personal philosophy.

main classifications in C. G. Jung's Psychological Types[2] differ in the general direction of interest. The introvert is chiefly concerned with the inner life; he tends to withdraw; he is diffident and not quite at home in the world of things and men. The opposite type, the extravert, turns mostly to the outside, is preoccupied with the world, the social life, and with activities operating in and upon the environment.

Another such division, proposed by G. Pfahler,[3] contrasts one type characterized by "rigidity of attention" with another of "fluid attention." There are several such typologies, but these two examples will suffice to show the formal nature of the differences discussed. The material content of the interest that turns inward or outward, of the attention that is rigid or fluid, is not considered. Yet one may well ask whether it does not make a definite difference in a man's conduct and in the structure of his personality whether, as an introvert, he is attracted by mathematics or by music; or, as an extravert, by sports or by engineering; whether he is more interested in the practice of politics or the study of experimental biology.

A typology that does consider the content rather than the form of mental activity, matter rather than manner, might be called material. Such is the typology first outlined by E. Spranger[4] and utilized, with some significant modifications, by G. Allport.[5] Here the psychological types are distinguished by the central values around which the individual's whole picture of reality is arranged. Such values may be those of abstract reason, of usefulness, of love, power, or religion. It is the person's main interest that is considered the distinctive trait in his being.

This same diversity of approaches occurs in the study of the prepsychotic personality: here, too, it is the formal approach that prevails. E. Kretschmer[6] has described the "schizoid" or "schizothymic" personality, of which the mental disease schizophrenia appears to be an intensification, and the opposite, "cycloid" or "cyclothymic" type – also

---

2 C. G. Jung, *Psychological Types* (New York, 1922).

3 G. Pfahler, "System der Typenlehren," *Beih. d. Zeitschr. f. Psychol.* (Leipzig, 1929), No. 15.

4 E. Spranger, *Lebensformen* (6th ed.; Halle a. s., 1927).

5 G. W. Allport, *Personality*, 2nd ed. (New York, 1939).

6 E. Kretschmer, *Physique and Character* (2nd ed.; London, 1936).

called "syntonic"[7] – in terms of strictly formal properties. Now it may be true that for an understanding of the relation between the pre psychotic mentality and the subsequent mental disease, the formal aspect is particularly relevant. We cannot, however, know whether or not this is the case until extensive inquiries have been made into the material aspect as well.

Descriptions of pre-morbid personalities in terms of Freudian psychoanalysis have made a certain contribution to the material aspect of the picture, but these, too, have largely been limited to formal considerations. They could hardly be otherwise, since it is the fundamental position of the psychoanalytic theory of human nature that man's goals are primarily those that promise satisfaction of instinctual needs; all other goals are seen as substitutes for these primary ones, and thus differences of material content lose their significance. The original purpose of psychoanalytic research was to discover the relation between neurotic states and the total life history of the individual, but in its later development it came increasingly to focus on the infantile stage. Now, the farther back the causes of neurotic symptoms are traced into the past of an individual, the less differentiated they appear, and at the infantile stage all values are reduced to the uniformity of immediate instinctual satisfaction where no differentiation is possible at all. The differences characterizing later stages of life are interpreted as a sort of superstructure erected on the ground of the primary instinctual needs; this superstructure may be of interest to a descriptive, but not to a genetic, approach.

It is an essential characteristic of psychoanalysis and almost all other types of medical psychology that the genetic viewpoint predominates. This emphasis is justified, since all medical practice seeks to remove disturbances by finding their causes and rendering them ineffective. It cannot, however, be assumed a priori that these causes will be found exclusively in the earliest periods of a man's life. Even if instincts and the fate they suffer in infancy are decisive factors, it is possible that their effects will depend on additional factors entering the picture at a later time. A predominant interest in such ultimate causes has prevented medical psychologists and psychiatrists from realizing the need to complement their inquiries with detailed descriptions of personali-

7 See, e.g., E. Minkowski, *La Schizophrénie, psychopathologie des schizoides et des schizophrènes* (new ed.; Paris, 1953).

ties and mental states, descriptions that take account of the material as well as formal factors determining conduct.

The formal characteristics of a personality, whether constitutional or arising from early experiences, exercise a definite influence on the material attitudes a person develops in his later life. They form the framework, as it were, within which all further experiences find their place and according to which they are interpreted. Since these factors are formal, however, their influence is by no means strict or inevitable. It allows for a wide variety of responses, and it can be largely modified, neutralized, or counterbalanced by other influences that come to bear on the individual after he has passed from the stage of unconscious and almost automatic reactions to that of conscious experience. Otherwise it would be impossible to understand why individuals develop into widely different personalities although the conditions of their infancy appear to have been the same. For instance, every child experiences frustration. If it is true that frustration often underlies aggressiveness, there must also be other factors at work, since not all children develop into aggressive, antisocial personalities.

It is, therefore, legitimate to ask whether, and to what extent, acquired attitudes, convictions, and general conceptions of reality may predispose toward, or modify, specific mental disturbances. One may put the question in this form: Are certain attitudes or world views more or less conducive than others to creating difficulties, engendering conflicts, making a man less capable of coming to terms with reality? Can one say that the chance of falling prey to mental disturbances is less for people who have acquired one set of convictions than for others whose convictions are of another, perhaps opposite, type?

APPROACHES TO AN ANSWER

These questions are not at all easy to answer. Today, some authors reject the idea of a causal relation between convictions and mental state and claim that it is rather the conviction that depends upon an actual or latent abnormal state. Others believe that there is a close interdependence between a man's convictions and principles, on the one hand, and his mental state or mental health, on the other. Both these arguments appear to be based much more on preconceived ideas than on an analysis of facts.

One might try to answer this question by means of a statistical survey. If it were found that mental disturbances were notably less frequent among people of one type of outlook or belief than among others, one might conclude that this particular outlook has certain protective powers. In fact, such attempts have been made, but they are not conclusive because of the enormous complexity of the cogent factors. For example, if certain religious beliefs are more frequent in one income bracket and less frequent in another, the incidence of mental illness among people holding those beliefs may be due to social rather than ideological factors. Moreover, it is difficult to assemble enough data for a reliable statistical elaboration. As N. Wiener[8] has pointed out, the "statistical runs" possible in social studies are much too short even to approach the accuracy of statistical physics. And finally, although a given number of people may say that they hold and live by certain beliefs, and although they may be perfectly sincere, one cannot know how closely their statements correspond to objective reality.

Even though statistics are not very helpful, however, there are certain data that strongly suggest a significant relation between mental health and a world view or philosophy, and there are certain inherent factors that make such a relation probable. Perhaps it is not a very strong argument, for example, but it is a fact that the incidence of mental disturbances, and especially of suicide, is remarkably low among philosophers.[9] Since their viewpoints vary so much, however, this would seem to suggest that the important thing is just to have any philosophy at all, to have worked it out and believe in it.

A more fundamental approach would be based on an analysis of human nature, and especially of cases in which an individual appears to resolve his difficulties when he attains greater clarity in matters of philosophy or of faith. In proceeding along these lines, however, it is extremely difficult to eliminate one's own bias, and there is always a danger of overrating the good influence of beliefs similar to one's own and the evil influence of others.

By the very nature of the psychotherapeutic process, a psychiatrist can never be perfectly certain that a cure has been the result of his

8 N. Wiener, *Cybernetics* (New York, 1951).

9 A rapid survey of the philosophers listed in Vol. IV of Ueberweg-Heinze's *Grundriss der Geschichte der Philosophie* (13th ed.; Basel, 1951) shows that among about 450 men who have lived and died in the period since 1800, there is one who became insane, Nietzsche (perhaps J. J. Rousseau is a second), and one who committed suicide, O. Weininger (who was not strictly a philosopher).

efforts, or certain of the role played by other co operating factors in bringing about a favorable result. The late Alfred Adler once remarked that half of all neurotics get well independently of the treatment they receive, simply because they have the will and ability to adopt a new attitude toward reality. In these instances the therapy becomes more of a "face saving" than a truly effective agent. Yet, even when the therapist believes that he has good reason for attributing a patient's recovery to his treatment, he still does not know for certain what the decisive influence was. He may claim that it was the unearthing of unconscious material, if he is a pupil of Freud; the awakening of the will of community, if he follows Adler; the force of persuasion, if he adopts the view of Dubois and others; but he cannot know for sure.

Other factors enter into every psychotherapeutic situation. Quite often the therapist is the first person, perhaps even since childhood, with whom the patient has established a human relation of some significance. He may be the only person with whom the patient can speak of things, not even necessarily personal or intimate, which he dares not or cannot mention to others. It does not matter in what terms this relation is described; call it "transference" if you wish, with all the implications of Freudian doctrine, or use some other name. The fact remains that in the therapeutic situation the isolation of the neurotic person is overcome, and the wall is broken through which had separated him from the world of his fellows and from reality.

Many psychiatrists will take these difficulties lightly and will consider the patient's recovery a sufficient proof both of the effectiveness of their treatment and the truth of their theories, but this is a fallacy. Human relations are much too complicated to permit such simple explanations. For the same reason, one cannot state that an individual's attitude has either caused or prevented an abnormal state, or that a change of attitude has caused an improvement in his condition. It is only in full awareness of the enormous complexity of all human affairs and of the need to avoid hasty generalizations that one may venture to approach the questions under consideration, propose certain tentative views, and try to support them by a careful analysis of the available facts.

II. PSYCHOTHERAPY & THE SCIENTIFIC METHOD

Science, which seeks to establish general laws, may and even must ignore individual differences. It is an essential feature of the experimental method that all individual circumstances be eliminated and that the phenomenon under investigation be made as "pure" as possible. From the viewpoint of medical science, each patient is a "case of – ." It is characteristic of a case that it fall under the general rule of its kind; it is an instance of a species, the manifestation of a general law. Just as every time an object falls to the floor the law of gravitation becomes manifest, and always does so in exactly the same way, so to medical science the case of pneumonia appears as one more manifestation of the general law that is called pneumonia.

In medical practice, however, one deals not with a controlled experiment, nor with an admixture of irrelevant, negligible factors, but rather with a sick person, and a person is the most individualized being of which we have knowledge. He is essentially unique; he is fundamentally not a "case" but an individual in his own right, unrepeatable. Thus, the practice of medicine has often been called an art rather than a science. Originally, the term *ars medica* meant simply that the activity of the physician consists in applying theoretical knowledge to practical use. *Ars*, the rendering of the Greek *téchne*, is the name for all practical disciplines and for the knowledge underlying them. It is significant, however, that this designation "art" has attained a specific connotation. It is generally understood to mean that mere knowledge, as acquired from books, lectures, and laboratory experience, is not enough, and that the physician must possess something more than theoretical knowledge. Theory deals with generalities, whereas art is concerned with particulars.

Medical practice must use an individualized approach because the patient's general attitude may influence the development of his illness, and also the extent of his co operation with the physician. The patient's individuality can "color" the disease, so that the pneumonia of Paul differs from that of Peter, even though both suffer from the same disease. On the other hand, the individuality of the patient may play a minor role when the question is whether or not to operate, and the choice of therapeutic procedures is almost independent of the patient's personality.

INDIVIDUALIZATION IN PSYCHIATRY

It is obvious that a person's response to illness depends largely on his general attitude; he may revolt; he may be reconciled; he may even welcome being an invalid and, therefore, "on leave," as it were. Yet one observes that notable changes in behavior are more likely to occur when the person's illness is one that involves all of himself rather than just, for example, a fractured leg. Even a slight infection such as the common cold may change a man's outlook. There are people who ought to be forbidden to make decisions while they have a cold or hay fever. Others will maintain a distance between themselves and their illness and consequently will be less affected in their relations with others and the world in general. Strictly speaking, neurosis is less a disease than a peculiar form of attitude toward reality or – to use an expression preferred today – toward existence. Because of the nature both of neurotic illness and of the curative procedures known as psychotherapy, individualization is much more important here than in other branches of medicine.

All treatment aims at the restoration of health, and health is a state of the whole man. When the physician treats a disturbed function, he aims, in truth, at the whole man. But his point of attack is only a part of the whole. Although it always deals with a diseased person and not just a diseased organ, medical treatment in the usual sense proceeds from the symptom or the disease hence, from a peripheral point, toward the ultimate aim of restoring normality to the whole human being.

The procedure of psychotherapy is fundamentally different from the procedures of all other branches of medicine.[10] The psychiatrist does not treat the neurotic heart as such, and he does not expect to restore normality by making the heart function normally. He expects that the normal functioning of the heart will occur when the total personality of the individual becomes normal. Thus, psychotherapy *proceeds from*

10 This does not mean, however, that psychotherapy is a mere technique or that the knowledge underlying it constitutes a discipline alien to medicine. The neurotic is fundamentally a sick person, though he suffers from a peculiar sickness, and dealing with him is essentially the task of a trained physician. This is particularly true since the diagnosis and treatment of many psychosomatic troubles require that the therapist be fully trained in medicine.

within, from the core of a man's being toward the peripheral manifestations.

It is here that the material factors discussed above require consideration, for the total being of a man cannot be described and understood in purely formal terms. To know what a person thinks, what preoccupies him, how things look to him, is at least as important for an adequate understanding of his being as to know that he is quick to anger, is given to incomprehensible changes of mood, or cannot shift his attention readily from one subject to another. If we are to understand a person, we must be familiar with his attitudes toward himself, toward things in general, and toward his fellow men.

One frequently encounters the statement that what is required is an "objective analysis" of a man's situation, meaning that all details of his situation should be carefully studied and listed. Even so, the resulting picture may he misleading. There may be features in the situation which seem quite outstanding to the observer but which are actually irrelevant because the subject does not consider them; they are simply nonexistent for him and consequently play no role in his life. On the other hand, features that appear negligible to the observer may have a marked significance for the subject, who sees them from a different angle. The situation which influences a man and to which he responds is not that revealed by objective analysis but that which he sees himself, and we shall not understand him until we can see things his way.[11]

CASE VS. PERSON

Science never reaches down to the individual but moves inevitably on the level of generalities. An approach that takes full account of individuality is no longer scientific, although it naturally uses all the help science may furnish. Basically, such an approach should be called *historical*. There is a slight recognition of this in the technical term "case history," except that one is dealing with the history not of a case but of a person. To repeat a statement I made many years ago: When the

11 Many so called incomprehensible actions on the part of normal or abnormal people can be understood in this way. The sudden refusal of a man to go any farther along a path becomes quite understandable once we know that he is very superstitious and that the black cat we hardly noticed was enough to make him change his plans. The same thing is true of the behavior of certain schizophrenics: little incidents that seem to us utterly insignificant may be full of portentous meaning to the schizophrenic.

physician leaves the laboratory and stands at the bed of a patient, he passes from a purely scientific approach to a historical one; he is confronted not simply with a case but with a person.[12]

It is interesting that case histories published by psychiatrists read very differently from those in medical journals and treatises. It has been said, not without reason, that the case histories written by disciples of Freud or Jung resemble modem novels, while those by followers of Adler are like moral tales. In any case, they are certainly more like biographies than anything else. This is only a superficial point, but it does indicate a significant difference between psychotherapy and other kinds of treatment. In any event, it has taken years for men of the various schools of psychotherapy to realize that neither the principles of medicine nor those of psychology in the usual sense are sufficient to cope with the problems encountered in psychotherapy.

The original intention of Breuer and Freud apparently involved some recognition of the fact that the problems they were studying required an approach other than that of scientific medicine. They obviously saw their problem to be that of integrating a person's life and experience, on the one hand, and the neurosis, on the other. The implicit shift away from a strictly medical and scientific viewpoint may have been one reason why psychoanalysis was rejected at first as unscientific. Disciples of Freud have pointed out that in recent years the charge has been reversed, and psychoanalysis is now criticized for being too scientific. The observation is justified, but it does not prove, as has been claimed, that opposition to Freud's theories is based not on any rational, experiential, or objective basis but on the "resistance" of those who cannot accept the theory because they have not personally undergone the experience of psychoanalysis. First of all, among the critics are some who have gone through analysis and were once orthodox Freudians. Secondly, psychoanalysis has not developed according to the plan implicit in the *Studies on Hysteria* of 1895, but, quite to the contrary, has sought to become as scientific as possible and to speak the language of science. Indeed, this tendency was also present from

---

12 R. Allers, "Begriff und Methodik der Deutung," in O. Schwarz, ed., *Psychogenese und Psychotherapie körperlicher Symptome* (Vienna, 1925). The German equivalent of case history is *Krankengeschichte* – that is, the history of a sick person; while the word is used largely in the same sense as case history, it can also be interpreted in the sense discussed here.

the beginning: Breuer and Freud gave their preliminary note the revealing title, "On the Mechanism of Hysterical Symptoms."

It should also be noted here that, partly because of the influence of Freud's thinking itself on all of the social sciences, and partly because of the great changes in the intellectual climate of Europe before and more particularly since World War I, the problems not only of psychotherapy but of all studies of man have appeared in a new light. It would be beyond the scope of this essay to attempt even a brief report of these intellectual developments, but it should be remembered that the present situation of psychotherapy is a part of this broader history of ideas.

Psychotherapists have gradually come to realize that even the life of a psychoanalytic patient involves something more than symptoms. It is understandable that a neurotic's ideas and problems may be seen as a part of his general, abnormal state, especially when they differ markedly from the physician's own convictions but this is, in fact, fallacious reasoning. The truth of a statement does not depend on the mental state of its maker. The proposition that two and two make four remains true even if a mentally disordered person says so; and it may well be the same with many other propositions. Moreover, the fact that a statement makes no sense to us does not prove that it is meaningless, for every mind has its limitations. We are all caught up in a network of preconceived ideas and thus prevented from seeing the truth, or even the possibility of it, in many statements that are alien to our habitual conceptual system.

The kind of mentality which has prevailed since the eighteenth-century Enlightenment and dominated the larger part of the nineteenth century has prevented the recognition of many problems. Even "today . . . psychologists write with the frankness of Freud or Kinsey on the sexual passions of mankind, but blush and grow silent when the religious passions come in view."[13] In so far as certain psychologists and psychiatrists consider such problems as religion at all, they view them as symptoms. They try to find out why a person is preoccupied with such questions, why they play a role in his life, and particularly what is "back of them" (their origin, in other words).

13 G. W. Allport, *The Individual and His Religion* (London, 1951), p. 1.

THE GENETIC FALLACY

Under the influence of psychoanalysis, modem psychology and psychiatry have fallen prey to what is known in logic as the "genetic fallacy" – that is, they confuse the discovery of origin with that of meaning.[14] This has two consequences, both of which have handicapped the understanding of neurosis and the development of an effective therapy in many cases. One of these consequences is the almost complete neglect of description or phenomenology. The statements of patients are taken at their face value, and no one asks whether two persons who speak of a feeling of guilt, for instance, actually mean the same thing. Quite possibly they do not. The second consequence is precisely that experiences are considered solely as manifestations of the origins from which they are supposed to have derived. The psychiatrist may be satisfied when, for instance, he has been able to trace a religious belief back to the Oedipus situation, or to interpret it as a mask for the will to superiority. He does not see any need to inquire into the present significance of the belief in his patient's life, much less its possible truth value.

It may, indeed, be characteristic of a certain person that he is preoccupied with a specific type of problem, but this fact does not imply any judgment on the problem itself.[15] It should be obvious that problems are not simply symptoms, and that they must be judged on the basis of

---

14 This confusion of origin and meaning has been pointed out recently by K. Jaspers, *Vernunft und Widervernunft im gegenwärtigen Philosophieren* (Munich, 1953). See also R. McKeon, *Thought, Action and Passion* (Chicago, 1954), p. 213: "We can explain aspects of the development of science, knowledge, and institutions ideologically, epistemologically, historically, and sociologically, but when we explain why men say what they do, we tend to discount what they mean when they say it."

15 We may note in passing that the same psychologistic and subjectivistic approach is found in those studies of art and poetry which are conceived according to psychiatric categories. One may well study the antecedents of a work of art, the personal experience of its creator, and even the "unconscious" material appearing in it, but all of this has nothing to do with the work as such, which must be judged for itself. In fact, knowledge of the artist's past and personality contributes nothing at all to a strictly aesthetic appreciation of the work or to an understanding of its meaning. The work speaks for itself and not for its maker. The psychogenic aspect is as irrelevant to a consideration of art or poetry as such as are, for instance, the details of the casting technique which Benvenuto Cellini used in making

their own intrinsic nature. Nevertheless, many medical psychologists still believe that it is improper for them, as psychologists, to deal with matters pertaining to religion, metaphysics, or the general world view of their patients, since such matters involve an element of value judgment which lies outside the scope of strictly scientific treatment.[16]

It is true, of course, that science does not and cannot consider values and, therefore, the motivations of individual actions. As H. Poincaré put it: "Science always speaks in the indicative, never in the imperative mood." The psychiatrist, however, expresses an evaluation the moment he speaks of someone as, for example, "maladjusted." The term implies not only that it is subjectively preferable to be adjusted, and thus to avoid suffering, conflicts, and social disturbance, but also that it is objectively better that people be adjusted to the conditions under which they have to exist.

Once they have grown roots, ideas do not die easily, and the persistent ideal of the scientific method is largely owed to what one might call cultural inertia. It was natural for a thinker trained in science and imbued with the nineteenth century idolatry of science to assume that all problems, including those of man's individual existence, could and would be solved by the appropriate scientific method. The demand that psychotherapy be primarily or even exclusively scientific, however, is born of prejudice and not imposed by the facts themselves. It deprives the psychotherapist of any possibility of seeing his patient's ideas and problems except as symptoms, or as irrelevant to the psychotherapeutic situation. When one stops to realize that ideas and attitudes are not mere superstructures but powerful agents, this position is quite untenable. Not only is the particular, the singular, beyond the grasp of scientific methodology, but the most important aspects of human existence, man's beliefs, his ideals, his ultimate motivations, all belong to a realm of reality with which science is unable to deal.

---

his Perseus, or the fact that Michelangelo's *Moses* consists of carbonate of calcium from Carrara.

16 See, for instance, Ch. Odier, *Les deux sources, consciente et inconsciente, de la vie morale* (Neufchatel, 1943); "À mon avis le concept d'autonomie, si psychologique soit il, est un concept limite au delà duquel le psychologue comme tel n'est pas fondé à s'aventurer. Il doit se borner à analyser et registrer les conditions de la restauration de cette autonomie, ou de la faculté d'accomplir un acte moralement libre."

The scientific method proceeds by analysis and seeks to reduce all phenomena to certain ultimate basic elements assumed to be constant and immutable, comparable to the atoms of a short time ago. In psychology these elements were "ideas" or "impressions," then "sensations," and more recently "instincts." The methodology of science requires that these basic elements and the laws governing their combination should suffice as principles of explanation. The world is reconstructed by putting together what analysis has separated. But this implies that only that can be integrated which analysis has been able to disengage from the complex whole of immediate experience. Since the elements are necessarily conceived of as being simple and, as it were, at the bottom of the scale of being, the resulting view is one that envisages things "from below."[17] Now there is no reason for assuming a priori that this view encompasses all of reality. Quite to the contrary, there is a strong presumption that this view leaves out certain most important factors. This is not to disclaim the usefulness and legitimacy of the procedure from below but simply to point out that it has not been and cannot be demonstrated to be universally and exclusively applicable.

III. THE CONTRIBUTION OF EXISTENTIALIST THOUGHT

The development of psychotherapy toward an increasing recognition of these problems runs parallel to a similar development in philosophy which has come to be known under the general heading of "existentialism."[18] In recent years there have been a number of writers who believe that real progress in the understanding and treatment of mental illness can be attained if psychiatry avails itself of the existentialist approach.

Among the philosophers, J. P. Sartre has written on "existential psychoanalysis,"[19] a term implying that psychoanalysis should consider the existential viewpoint. There are also some incidental references to

17 For a further discussion of the "view from below" and that "from above," see Allers, *The New Psychologies* (London–New York, 1931).

18 The best survey and analysis of these philosophies is that in J. Collins, *The Existentialists* (Chicago, 1952).

19 J. P. Sartre, *L'Etre et le néant* (Paris, 1943). See also A. Stern, *Sartre, His Philosophy and Psychoanalysis* (New York, 1953).

psychiatric problems in the writings of Gabriel Marcel.[20] Among psychiatrists, L. Binswanger was probably the first to study the problems of psychotherapy in the light of the philosophy of M. Heidegger,[21] a writer who has influenced several contemporary psychiatrists. Following Heidegger's terminology, Binswanger speaks of *Daseinsanalyse,* a term difficult to translate because Dasein means not simply "existence" but the kind of existence proper to man. Binswanger seems to believe that something like an analysis of existence is possible. Since 1934 V. E. Franki has advocated an approach with a similar name, *Existenzanalyse,* but he actually seeks not to analyze existence but to envisage an "existential" form of life as the goal of psychotherapy.[22] I. Caruso proposes the "psychoanalysis of existence" and even the "synthesis of existence," as does his pupil, W. Daim.[23] One must beware of being confused by these very similar terms, for the ideas they represent are actually quite diverse. One may also question whether some of these terms, for instance, "psychoanalysis of existence" and "synthesis of existence," can be used significantly at all. Laxity of expression is apt to lead to inaccuracy of thinking.

A QUESTION OF METAPHOR

An even more dangerous pitfall is that of the metaphor. It is too easily forgotten that most of the terms used in psychology and psychiatry are metaphors and do not directly indicate the nature of that to which they refer. Through frequent use they come to be taken as denotations of reality. Thus it is customary to refer to certain schools of psychotherapy by the common name of "depth psychology" and to speak of "depths" or "layers" of the human mind. This seems to be a natural metaphor, since common parlance includes such expressions as "deeply moved," a "superficial" state, and others. Yet it is not a metaphor common to all languages; ancient Greek, for example, spoke of a "deep" emotion as a "heavy" one. However much the metaphor of depth may

20 R. Troisfontaines, *De l'existence à l'être: La philosophie de Gabriel Marcel* (Paris, 1953).

21 L. Binswanger, *Ausgewählte Vorträge und Aufsätze* (Berne, 1947). See the new treatise by U. Sonnemann, *Existence and Therapy* (New York, 1954).

22 V. E. Frankl, *Ärztliche Seelsorge* (Vienna, 1946), and *Der unbewusste Gott* (Vienna, 1948).

23 I. Caruso, *Psychoanalyse und Synthese der Existenz* (Vienna, 1952). W. Daim, *Umwertung des Psychoanalyse* (Vienna, 1951).

suggest, it remains a metaphor, and one is not entitled to speak of the "layers" of the mind as realities.

Neither language nor imagination possesses adequate means for referring to mental or ideal things, and the use of metaphor is inevitable. Nevertheless, it is misleading to say, as is regularly said, that Freud "discovered" the unconscious, or repression, or regression, or anything else. Actually, Freud made certain observations the novelty and originality of which no one will contest, and he invented certain names, that is, metaphors, as convenient ways to refer to these discoveries. In the same way, no one has ever observed an instinct; the term is a convenient label and hypothetical explanation for a definite kind of behavior observed with great regularity in certain animal species.[24]

If one remembers the metaphorical character of psychological terminology, and realizes also that philosophy must depend upon metaphorical terminology,[25] one will not so readily see a confirmation in the coincidence of terms used in the two fields. A philosophy that has derived its terms chiefly from physics and mechanics, for example, will sound like the findings of a psychiatrist who uses the same metaphors. It may be, however, that all the two have in common is terminology, and it is even possible that both have chosen metaphors that could be replaced by others better suited to deal with the facts. Thus a careful and searching consideration of metaphors and, indeed, of all terms is necessary. A survey of the writings called "existentialist," for example, leads one to the conclusion that the very term "existence" means different things to different thinkers, and that we may not borrow one statement on existence from one writer, and a second statement from another, without ascertaining what their respective positions are.

---

24 It is instructive to experiment with the devising of other metaphors to replace those currently in use. The metaphor of depth, for instance, can he replaced by that of center and periphery. Repression then becomes expulsion; the unconscious is not deep down but far out. This metaphor may be developed in detail, and in doing so one realizes how many of our ideas about the operations of the mind are dependent on the metaphor, and how different things can look when the metaphor is changed.

25. The source of a philosopher's fundamental metaphors makes a difference to his total outlook. This can be seen clearly if one compares philosophies inspired by Plato-Plotinus-St. Augustine with those whose lineage is that of Aristotle-St. Thomas Aquinas.

Once these qualifications have been noted, however, there is no doubt that the existentialist movement has brought to the fore problems of immediate concern to the psychologist and, perhaps even more, to the psychiatrist. Philosophers are not psychologists, but what they have to say is often extremely useful to the psychologist, and this modern movement is certainly closer to human reality than were many philosophies of the past. In spite of their differences, all the existentialist philosophies share a common concern for the being of the individual person as such, in the concrete situation of his life. Since his being, or its manifestation, is codetermined by the situation, which in turn must be seen as it is experienced rather than as it is objectively given, it appears that the reversal of Fichte's proposition is justified – that the kind of man one is does depend on one's philosophy or attitude toward the world.

BEING-IN-A-WORLD

Heidegger's fundamental notion is that man is inevitably, by virtue of his very being, in a world. Being in a world is a constitutive factor of man's existence. But this world takes on a new aspect each time it is viewed by another person. The problems to be dealt with are not those of ontology, which would consider the being of man in general and his world in general; the problems concern "factually occurring forms and configurations of existents."[26] The relevance of this approach for psychotherapy is obvious. Because of this viewpoint, existentialists criticize other philosophies as "essentialistic" – that is, as dealing with the general nature or essence of man. Existential analysis (a term much to be preferred to "analysis of existence") does not seek to discover causal relations or the origin of this or that phenomenon; it seeks "the spiritual (*geistig*) connection between the contents of experience."[27]

Although this formulation of being in a world is peculiar to Heidegger, and he particularly emphasizes this aspect of human existence, the ego's concern with the non ego is central in all the existentialist philosophies.[28] When man encounters the world, or his world, he is forced by the very dynamics of his being to seek an interpretation of

26 L. Binswanger, *op. cit.*, p. 190.

27 *Ibid.*, p. 61.

28. This is particularly true of Gabriel Marcel. See Sonnemann, *op. cit.*, p. 126.

what he encounters. And let it be noted once more that the truth or falsity, adequacy or inadequacy, of such interpretations does not depend on the way man arrives at them. All merely genetic analysis is absolutely powerless before actual questions about life, its significance, man's place in the order of things, and his ultimate destiny. Thus the new ideas emphasize the importance of problems that the psychotherapy of the last half century has either disregarded or treated as mere symptoms. Although the two new Viennese schools, those of V. E. Frankl and I. Caruso, must not be confused, they do both speak of existence and stress the relevance of religion for human life and for the re establishment of satisfactory relations between the individual and reality.

It may be asked why there has been no mention here of the ideas of C. G. Jung. The Swiss psychiatrist has often been regarded as one who, going beyond the teachings of his master Freud, has given full recognition to the role religion plays and ought to play in human life. A closer examination reveals, however, that Jung's views differ considerably from those of the Viennese schools and certainly from those of any truly religious person. He is not concerned with the truth value of religion or with the metaphysical questions involved. In Jung's "complex psychology" God is not a transcendent reality of which man may achieve some knowledge by means of natural reason, but rather an "archetype" or externalization of a basic tendency in human nature.[29] The ideas of God, of divine justice, of a future life, and all the other tenets of religion are seen not as expressing reality but as corresponding to a subjective need. Jung has not gone beyond the subjectivism so eminently characteristic of the nineteenth century mentality.

SYMBOLS AND SUBJECTIVISM

This subjectivism is evident in Jung's whole theory of archetypes. He had observed – a most interesting and important observation, indeed – that certain figures of an obviously symbolic nature[30] occur in quite different civilizations and are also produced in spontaneous drawings by people who know nothing of cultural anthropology or comparative religion. According to his way of thinking, the only possible explana-

29. For a different interpretation, see V. White, *God and the Unconscious* (Chicago, 1953).

30 On the meaning of the term "symbol," see below.

tion is that these images dwell somehow, hidden from ordinary consciousness, in every man's mind; they are archetypes not of reality but of mental operations. It did not occur to him that in fact one can, and probably with better reason, explain the recurrence of symbols as the result of objective rather than subjective factors.

It may be helpful here to consider some similar ideas that play a prominent role in psychoanalytic theory, those of "regression," and of "archaic" and "magical' thinking. Freud believed in a definite parallelism between the development of the individual mind and that of the mind of mankind as manifested in the history of civilization. He applied here the so called "law of ontogenesis" formulated by E. Haeckel, which states that the development of the individual organism recapitulates, in an abbreviated manner, the development of the race. Now, even if Haeckel's law is assumed to be valid, this does not necessarily justify Freud's application of it, for there is an enormous difference between the history of the race and the growth of civilization. The first involves the operation of natural forces over many geological periods, while the second has to do with man's own activities during a relatively brief period.[31] Freud's application appeared conceivable because of the metaphorical use of the term "development," and it expressed his fundamental belief that all human operations must be of the same basic nature as those of forces in the physical universe. Various facts have been used to support the theory, even though they do not demonstrate it.[32]

Freud's theory appeared to be confirmed by the writings of L. Lévy-Bruhl, published in 1910.[33] According to this author, the primitive

31 Even so convinced a naturalistic thinker as Julian Huxley realizes that with the appearance of man and the beginnings of civilization factors became effective other than those which determine phylogenesis. See J. Huxley, *Evolution* (New York, 1941), especially the concluding pages.

32 This is one of the many instances of circular reasoning which one discovers in the theories of Freud, See R. Allers, *The Successful Error* (New York, 1940). See also, V. Sonnemann, *op. cit.*, p. 163. Orthodox Freudians, however, refuse to recognize even the demonstration of factual errors. In 1946 in a lecture at the Sorbonne, Anna Freud still maintained that "the child is born in the Stone Age and has to attain, within five years, the actual civilization." Quoted by A. Stocker, *Psychologie du sens moral* (Geneva, 1948), p. 178.

33 L. Lévy-Bruhl, *Les fonctions mentales dans les sociétés inférieures*, (Paris, 1910).

mind functions in a different manner from that of civilized man. He declared that the principle of contradiction has no place in primitive thinking, which is dominated by the "law of participation;" it is "magical thinking" and is "pre logical." Severely criticized by both cultural anthropologists and psychologists, Lévy-Bruhl gradually moderated his more extreme statements, and at the end of his life he was preparing a book that was altogether to retract his previous views.[34] He frankly admitted that "pre logical" thought does not exist; that the principles governing the thinking of primitives were the same as our own; that the whole idea of a development from magical to realistic and finally to scientific ways of thinking was a fictitious construct.

This retraction failed to impress the psychoanalysts, and those psychiatrists who followed their lead.[35] They still cling to the notion of archaic thinking as the only possible explanation for similarities observed in the thinking of primitives, infants, and schizophrenics, This explanation is based on the concept of regression and assumes that under the impact of mental illness or of a shock suffered in encountering a reality with which the individual cannot come to terms, the mind retreats to a more primitive stage, one that it had already passed through, individually, in the development from infancy to adulthood, and racially, in the progress from primitive to advanced civilization. Because of the prevailing subjectivist trend, this appeared to be the only possible explanation.

Once subjectivism is abandoned and the idea of being in the-world is taken seriously, another approach becomes possible. Obviously human nature has not changed fundamentally since its earliest times.[36] Men respond to similar situations in a similar way; if they did not, we could understand neither our fellow men nor history. No particularly penetrating analysis is required to realize that primitives, infants,

34 Les carnets de Lucien Lévy-Bruhl (Paris, 1951). For a more detailed discussion, see R. Allers, "Über die Begriffe eines archaischen Denkens und der Regression," *Wiener Zeitschrift für Nervenheilkunde*, I (1941), 287.

35 They had given no consideration to the critical remarks of such men as the eminent cultural anthropologist B. Malinowski, or G. Cassirer, whose views are summarized in his *Essay on Man* (New Haven, 1948), esp. p. 80.

36 On primitives, see W. Koppers, "Lévy-Bruhl und das Ende des 'praelogischen' Denkens," Reprint: *Abhandl. d. 14 Internat. Soziologen Kongr.*, IV, Rome, 1951.

and schizophrenics all live in similar worlds: they are thrown into a world of which they are largely ignorant, confronted by strangeness and by unaccountable, unpredictable events, exposed to dangers they cannot foresee, and made victims of forces they cannot control. It is certainly understandable that their responses should all be more or less the same.

The same approach can be used to consider the recurrence of symbols which Jung sought to explain. It is conceivable that certain common data of experience and certain forms and shapes that come readily to mind are, by their own nature, symbols; they reveal a "world of meaning." In other words, symbols are not so much created as discovered. Both natural phenomena and artifacts may prove to be symbolic in themselves. One of the commonest symbols is the wheel, and another is the door. Both are artifacts and were certainly not invented as symbols.

RELIGION AND SCIENTIFIC NEUTRALITY

When subjectivism is abandoned, psychotherapy must become seriously concerned with the objective referents of subjective states, for these states are seen to be the responses of the individual to the world as he encounters it. Metaphysical and religious matters cannot be regarded merely as symptoms. It is not enough to know, (if it can be known) what factors determine a man's concern with such problems; the problems themselves must be understood. Nor is it enough to introduce a "religious instinct" among other instincts, for such a hypothetical, and highly questionable, notion brings us no nearer to the problem."[37] An instinct, it seems, is an innate tendency enabling the organism to cope with certain aspects of reality or to function in certain concrete situations as they occur in the life of the species. To speak of a religious instinct implies, if the term is to make sense at all, that such matters form part of reality. Naturally, it is not at all the intention of the subjectivist psychologists to admit this.

However religion may be interpreted, the recognition that psychotherapy must deal with such matters raises serious problems. The

37 V. E. Frankl (*Des unbewusste Gott*, p. 96), in a passage that contains an incisive criticism of Jung's subjectivist notions, refers to a statement by H. Bänziger (*Schweizer Zeitschrift für Psychologie*, VI, 1947, p. 281): "One may speak of a religious instinct (*Trieb*) as of a sexual instinct or an instinct of aggression."

therapist can no longer rely on mere technique and maintain the aloofness he has claimed as his right and, indeed, as the necessary condition of his activity; inevitably, he is personally engaged. If he believes, in one way or another, in a transcendent or supernatural reality, then he may intentionally or unintentionally try to persuade his patient to adopt his views. In fact, this happens easily and not infrequently even with those psychologists who believe that they are "neutral" and harbor no such beliefs at all. In the matter of philosophical or religious world views, no neutrality is possible. What is often called neutrality is a kind of tolerance for beliefs that are felt to be arbitrary or superstitious or incompatible with science and reason. But even tolerant indifference and scepticism are also beliefs of a kind, and the most tolerant person may involuntarily influence another's way of thinking, especially in the peculiar relationship that develops in psychotherapy. Just a simple inquiry on the part of the psychiatrist – "Is that what you believe?" – may be enough to make the patient feel uncertain of his convictions, and thus may become the source of conflicts sometimes more serious than those for which he sought help in psychotherapy.

It cannot be the task of the psychotherapist to "convert" his patient. However strong his convictions and however good his reasons for them, they have no place in the psychotherapeutic situation as such. If some belief of a more or less religious nature should prove necessary for the patient's return to normality and a satisfactory form of existence, a truly neutral formula must be found which is independent of the convictions of psychiatrist and patient alike, that is, a definition of the "minimum requirements" to be met.

Some people, of strong and sharply defined religious convictions, feel that to limit oneself to such minimum requirements would be an improper compromise. Anything less than the whole truth, as they see it, appears almost equivalent to falsehood, for if one knows the truth, he has an obligation to proclaim it. Understandable as this viewpoint may be, it is both unfounded in theory and untenable in practice. These overzealous folk would do well to reflect on the words of St. Paul about the milk to be given to infants and the solid food suitable for adults. The minimum requirements should be such that they are acceptable to everyone) whatever his religious training, whatever his attitudes and prejudices.

OPEN FROM ABOVE

"To many people a sense of cosmic affiliation is needed Love of Cod is needed in order to make life seem complete, intelligible, and right."[38] Indeed, man's existence is not fully characterized by Heidegger's formula of being in a world, for this world and man's existence are, so to speak, open from above. They require some sort of fulfillment. It is not possible to demonstrate with the cogency of a chemical formula or mathematical equation – the tenets of orthodox Christianity. Still less can nontheological science cope with the more or less undefined "cosmic affiliation" Allport posits. But reason, when it is not held back by too many prejudices, can and frequently does bring people far along toward discovery of theological truth.

The most powerful obstacles to thought about religion are fears of not being sufficiently modern, advanced, or in step with science. The so called advanced mind criticizes the faithful, and those who find meaning in metaphysical speculation, for harboring "obsolete" views. This same advanced mind seems to be utterly unaware of the fact that it is simply repeating the rather shopworn ideas of the eighteenth century Enlightenment. The student of the history of ideas is sometimes amazed at the naïveté with which ideas are presented as new which were actually put forward by *les philosophes* and their followers.

Comparable is the position of E. Fromm, who holds that religion, especially when represented by an ecclesiastical organization, is necessarily "authoritarian" and, therefore, to be rejected in favor of the independence and self responsibility of the human person.[39] Fromm fails to make two important distinctions. He confuses a voluntary and responsible acceptance of faith with the immature submissiveness of an underdeveloped mind. And he confuses the authority of office with that of truth. Actually, when one believes that a doctrine is true, he submits to it by the same inherent necessity that compels him to accept a mathematical proposition, even though the assent is of a somewhat different character. But the "faithful" recognize that certain dogmatic and moral precepts are in harmony with the demands of reason and conscience *simultaneously* with their recognition that the teaching and legislating Church, having its authority from God, cannot possibly profess doctrines or impose laws that would be unreasonable or

38 G. W. Allport, *op. cit.*, p. 91.

39 E. Fromm, *Escape from Freedom* (New York, 1941).

unconscionable. The mature believer accepts the tenets of his Faith with the same free, intelligent assent with which he agrees to obey its laws, and with the same justification: the divine *reason* of divine *power*. Truth sets man free.

Similarly, it cannot be said that conscience is a product of parental authority, a remnant of the infantile situation which still burdens the individual and which he obeys as he once obeyed his parents[40]. This is a case where generalizing from the observation of abnormal personalities (as is done in contemporary psychology) proves a hindrance to the adequate understanding of the phenomenon in question. The practice of assuming that the characteristics observed in abnormal personalities are common to all men is based ultimately on the idea that such phenomena as conscience are without objective reality anyway and must be seen as symptoms of something else.

SYMBOLS ARE NOT SYMPTOMS

This is often overlooked because discussions of such mailers are likely to be in terms of symbols rather than symptoms. Now there is a great deal of difference between the two: the symptom is caused by the underlying trouble, but the symbol does not owe its existence to that which it symbolizes. Freud, however, considered a symbol to be a kind of symptom and thus confused two totally different relations, that of causation and that of signification.[41] A symptom indicates and permits the discovery of some delimited trouble; a symbol refers to a context of meaning which becomes manifest, though not necessarily perfectly clear, to the subject.

The hasty identification of symptom and symbol is one of the features of psychoanalysis which recent work seeks to eliminate. Binswanger

40 G. W. Allport, *op. cit.*, p. 100: "Conscience in the normal personality may not be considered as a carry over from childhood, a parentally imposed superego."

41 I have remarked above that this identification is unfounded. It was possible because of the fact that in psychoanalysis when a symptom is traced back to its origin, as that is understood in Freud's doctrine, the symptom disappears. Freud saw this as an experiential confirmation of his view. However, it is not possible to generalize from such observations to a theory which will be valid in all instances, even those in which experiential confirmation is unattainable. In the case of an analyzed dream, for example, the analyzed dream element cannot disappear because it has disappeared already.

with his notion of *Daseinsanalyse*, Sartre when he speaks of *psychanalyse existentielle*, Frankl in attempting to complement psychotherapy by "logotherapy," Caruso with his idea of analysis of existence – all realize that one is dealing not simply with symbol symptoms but with the manifestation of the total being of a human person.[42] Although Caruso's term "synthesis of existence" is of questionable nature, because that which by definition is an organic whole cannot be put together or synthesized from an assortment of elements or parts, the idea does involve a recognition that analysis is not enough, that the interpretation of human life involves more than breaking it down into relationships between elementary constitutive factors such as Freud's instincts.

There are profound differences among the various existentialist philosophies which cannot be considered here, but they all have in common a serious concern with the understanding of man as an individual living in the world, and a belief that previous philosophies have failed to provide adequate means for reaching such an understanding.[43] In the course of their work, the existentialist schools have accumulated an amazing amount of empirical material. Their approach is neither that of the psychology taught and practiced in modern laboratories nor that of medical psychology as it has grown out of the ideas of Freud and others. It is a "phenomenological" psychology, which attempts to describe precisely what goes on in a man living in a definite situation. It recognizes that the situation to which a man responds must be understood as it appears to him, through the medium of his own fundamental attitude toward reality. And reality here means not simply the environment but everything outside the ego – the whole universe of things and events, of institutions and ideas, of facts and values, including the person himself.

42 "The principle of this psychoanalysis (existential) is that man is a totality and not a collection; that, consequently, he expresses himself totally even in the most superficial and most insignificant conduct." J. P. Sartre, *L'Etre et le néant* (Paris, 1948), p. 656.

43 For a pertinent criticism of non phenomenological psychologies and their significance, or lack of significance, for an understanding of man's being or existence, see the discussion of behaviorism and configurationalism (*Gestaltpsychology*) in Sonnemann's book, *passim*.

IV. TOWARD A FULLER UNDERSTANDING OF THE HUMAN SITUATION

Out of recent trends in philosophy on the one hand, and certain inherent difficulties of psychotherapy on the other, there has arisen a recognition of the role played by a person's world view in his individual existence. The implications of this new understanding, when recognized in their full significance, will undoubtedly transform the current ideas of psychotherapy. The situations both of the psychotherapist and of his patient will appear in a new light.

The medical, analytic, scientific approach that has prevailed until now has tended to regard all mental troubles, whether they were diseases in the strict sense or conflicts, as something which "happens" to the individual. Accordingly, the patient is an almost wholly passive object of therapeutic efforts. He is expected to cooperate to some extent, but fundamentally the cure "happens" to him just as the development of a neurosis happened. Today, however, it is "not unrealistic to think that a man is capable of being responsible for himself."[44] It is possible to see a man's personality not simply as the product of innate disposition fashioned by environmental forces, but as something which he himself has achieved and which, therefore, he may also transform. Of course, an individual's potentialities are limited by the given nature of his being, but within these limits there is room for a great variety of developments depending to a large extent on man's own choice. Personality is not given but entrusted to man.[45] The motto of the new schools in psychotherapy might well be the words uttered first by Pindar, repeated by Plotinus, and taken up by Goethe: "Become thou what thou art."

MINIMUM REQUIREMENTS AGAIN

In any case, whatever a man may be by virtue of his uniqueness as a person, he partakes of human nature and shares with others the human situation. The question therefore arises whether there may be some general outline of human personality and human conduct within which man must move if he is to avoid serious conflicts with himself

44 A. Roe, "The Use of Clinical Diagnostic Technique in Research with Normals," in *Feelings and Emotions: The Mooseheart Symposium*, ed. M. L. Reymert (New York, 1950), p. 341.

45 R. Allers, *Self Improvement* (New York, 1939).

and the world around him. We return to the question of minimum requirements[46] – a question that is so complex and involves so many problems that even to outline it and to suggest, not an answer but the way to look for an answer, is very difficult. While it is certainly true that a "right ordering of life" may prevent conflicts and neuroses, it is far from easy to say in what such a right ordering consists.[47]

The term "minimum requirement" may be taken to mean two things that are related but nevertheless distinct. It may mean, first, man's minimum requirements for subsistence. As there are physical conditions that must be met for life to be preserved, and others, before life deserves to be called human, so there are other kinds of conditions which must be met before man can live without too heavy a burden of conflicts and too much dissatisfaction. Sociologists and psychologists have spoken of "basic needs" the nonfulfillment of which depresses man's life below the minimum level, but these basic needs cannot be defined in biological terms. Georg Simmel has remarked that life demands not only more life but more than life; and Ortéga y Gasset has pointed out that satisfaction of the vital needs is not enough to render a life a human life.[48] Moreover, what is required beyond the fulfillment of strictly vital needs varies considerably with individuals, civilizations, and social circumstances. An effort to define minimum requirements in this more elementary sense encounters great difficulties.

Secondly, the term "minimum requirements" may refer not to the demands man makes on the world, but to the demands the world makes on him. It is here that very serious problems arise, for it is customary to include the various troubles and conflicts making up a neurosis under the general concept of maladjustment, and then to regard the task

46 The question discussed here also has definite implications for the role of the psychiatrist. "Good and bad are essentially ethical concepts and have no place in the realm of science . . . To the psychiatrist, however, . . . a maladjustment is an ailment to be treated . . . he is called upon not only to investigate but also to judge and to modify behavior." L. F. Shaffer, *The Psychology of Adjustment* (Boston, 1936), p. 137.

47 ". . . psychotherapists today are inclined to forget that a right ordering of life which is fully accepted and acted upon prevents conflicts and, therefore, neurosis." M. B. Arnold, "The Theory of Psychotherapy," in M. B. Arnold and J. A. Gasson, *The Human Person* (New York, 1958), p. 531.

48 G. Simmel, *Lebensanschauung* (Munich, 1918). J. Ortéga y Gasset, *Toward a Philosophy of History*, trans. H. Weyl (New York, 1941).

of the psychotherapist as that of reconstituting the individual's adjustment to his situation. This approach fails to consider the question of whether adjustment to actually prevailing conditions is always to be equated to normality and will always eliminate disturbances and bring about a greater capacity for activity and for enjoyment.

ADJUSTMENT – TO WHAT?

In fact, it is quite possible that the conditions to which a person is expected to adjust are such that conformity would cause even greater troubles than those of maladjustment. And I am not referring here to conditions so extreme and unusual as to make demands beyond the limits of human tolerance. Paradoxical as it may sound, it may be normal, or at least healthy, for an individual to respond abnormally to highly abnormal situations. To be adjusted or to try to achieve adjustment to certain conditions might be more harmful than helpful in the effort to work out a tolerable form of existence. Modern man sometimes finds himself forced to live with a certain group and to conform to the group pattern. If he refuses to conform, he will be ostracized. Yet the group pattern may be contrary to the deepest tendencies of his being, and conformity may make demands on him which will sooner or later become intolerable and cause serious conflicts within himself. For such a person, no course of action can ensure a normal form of existence.

One may call these developments unfortunate; nevertheless they are real, and no individual can change them. A psychiatrist may firmly believe in the need of every individual to be wholly himself within the limits of possibility and may realize that the straight jacket of a group pattern threatens to suffocate the very being of his patient. The patient may see clearly that most of his conflicts would disappear under different circumstances. Neither can do anything about the situation. It is a fact that too many persons find themselves caught in situations from which they are unable to extricate themselves.[49] Thus it is almost impossible to define minimum requirements because they would still not ensure a satisfactory form of existence where external conditions prevent it. Moreover, individuals differ, and a situation that is toler-

49 V. E. Frankl is certainly right in saying that "one becomes a man in the true sense only at the point where he is free to resist the sort of determinism which produces types (*Ärztliche Seelsorge*, p. 58). But how can he be free to do so?

able for one may be felt as beyond the limits of tolerance by another. Some people find compensations for an unsatisfactory existence in an intense religious life, or intellectual avocations, or artistic activity; others have no such resources.

The discontent caused by the emptiness and mechanization of modern life[50] has given rise to the demand that man have an opportunity to "express himself." It is certainly true that sell expression gives some help, but it is not enough, especially over a long period of time. For self expression to be significant, there must be something in the self which seeks and deserves expression. The expression of an empty self is but an empty gesture. What man really seeks, when he clamors for self expression, is something else. The real trouble is that his life is devoid of significance and he is incapable of creative achievement. The consequence of this tragic situation is that man is more and more concerned with receiving, less and less with giving. Emptiness, it seems, must be filled from without; hence, man becomes more and more demanding and is haunted by the fear of not getting enough.

One might go on indefinitely describing the unfortunate entanglement in which modern man has allowed himself to be caught, but even this brief discussion is sufficient to indicate that easy solutions and simple formulae are unattainable. Moreover, the problem is the more difficult since even under the equalizing conditions of modern existence man does not cease to be an individual in the strictest sense of the term. At the same time, it is true that the uniqueness of a human being is increasingly blurred as he is less himself and, therefore, farther from normality. All abnormality is in some sense a diminution or defect, and therefore is destructive of individuality. The more abnormal a man becomes, the more he will be "true to type," and idiots and the demented insane retain little if any individuality qua human beings. A study of man which starts from that of abnormal people is, therefore, always exposed to the danger of overlooking essential aspects of man's being.[51]

---

50 Cf. G. Marcel, Man against Humanity (London, 1952), and D. Riesman, N. Glazer and R. Denney, The Lonely Crowd (New Haven, 1950). The American edition of the Marcel work is titled Man against Mass Society (Chicago, 1952).

51 B. Bosanquet once remarked that human nature can be studied better in the great heroes, geniuses, and saints of history than in the inmates of men-

Whatever the circumstances of man's existence, it seems that it may be possible to reach a sufficient understanding of his nature to establish certain conditions as necessary for the achievement of a normal and satisfactory existence. We must not, however, delude ourselves into believing that the fulfillment of necessary conditions will ensure success. Without them, the goal cannot be attained, but with them one can still fail.

For the achievement of a world view that takes account of being in its totality, it is evident that the fundamental condition is the acceptance of man's place in the order of being, the attitude that Gabriel Marcel has appropriately termed "ontological humility."[52] In Heidegger's conception of being in the world as the fundamental characteristic of man's station something similar is implied, but it is not developed to the same extent as in Marcel. We have seen that Heidegger's ideas have exercised a considerable influence on psychiatrists whose approaches are otherwise as different as those of Binswanger, Frankl, and Caruso. On the other hand Marcel's conceptions – which ought to be of considerable interest to Christian psychiatrists – have attracted little if any attention. There are in Marcel's works many views and observations that psychotherapy could utilize.[53]

Neither Heidegger nor Marcel is specifically concerned with the problems of psychiatry, but J. P. Sartre has devoted a chapter of his main philosophical work to a discussion of "existential psychoanalysis." While this is not the place to discuss either Sartre's philosophy or his ideas on psychoanalysis,[54] a few brief comments will serve to introduce our final considerations.

---

tal hospitals and prisons. *The Value and Destiny of the Individual* (London, 1918).

52 G. Marcel, *Being and Having*, trans. K. Farrer (London, 1949).

53 1 owe my acquaintance with this thinker's work to the unpublished master's dissertation of my student Miss Guillemine de Vitry, whom I wish to thank here for permission to use her essay.

54 For a critical analysis of Sartre's ideas, see A. Stern, *Sartre, His Philosophy and Psychoanalysis* (New York, 1953), and more recently, W. Desan, *The Tragic Finale. An Essay on the Philosophy of Jean Paul Sartre* (Cambridge, 1954).

THE TWO WAYS OPEN TO MAN

When man realizes, not only theoretically but with the whole of his being, what his nature is – that of a finite being with infinite possibilities – there seem to be two ways open to him. One way is that of self aggrandizement, the insensate attempt to raise himself to the level of an absolute. He then falls into despair, as Kierkegaard so clearly saw. This despair may not be recognized by the subject and may be disguised in many forms, one of which is precisely neurosis.[55] Sartre's atheistic existentialism is the imposing but hopeless attempt to make this fundamentally abnormal state the norm of human existence.

The other way is that of faith. This is the way of Gabriel Marcel. But a faith that is capable of transforming man's being must be more than the acceptance of certain tenets and the fulfillment of certain obligations. It must become one with the person's being.

Sartre writes that man's most profound desire, the very source of all his doing and striving, is to become God. He seems unaware of the fact that Alfred Adler saw in this striving precisely one of the basic traits of the neurotic character. It probably means nothing to the author of this tragic atheistic existentialism that his words sound amazingly like the tempting and deluding promise of the Serpent. What Sartre asks is certainly not "minimum requirements." His philosophy is one of despair because it is one of absurdity: since he cannot explain why things are, and why they are as they are, he judges the whole realm of being to be absurd. Indeed, his ideas constitute a "tragic finale," as W. Desan aptly calls it – but if so, it is a tragedy without catharsis. It leaves man in the depths of hopelessness, and the only consolation it offers him is the assurance that the little meaning he may find in life will be his own work.

For all the subtleties of his analysis, Sartre's picture of man is pitiably incomplete. The success his work has found is understandable at a time when most men feel unable to make sense of their situation and unable to find a place for themselves. It is not that they cannot exist within society, or that the serious defects of modem society cannot be remedied. They find no place because they no longer know what they are.

---

55 I pointed out as far back as 1929 that "at the bottom of every neurosis there is a metaphysical problem." *The Psychology of Character*, trans. E. B. Strauss (London–New York, 1931).

The finite can be understood only against the background of the infinite. The image can be understood only when seen as a reflection of the original. To understand himself man will have to realize anew, and with the totality of his being, that he is made in the image and likeness of his Creator. But religion and conscientious compliance with the obligations of the Faith are not enough; these are but the necessary conditions. Man must be made capable of living his faith. Instead of striving for adjustment, he must strive for being; instead of seeking more and more goods, he must seek to become good himself.

It is not the task of psychotherapy either to convert its patients or to indoctrinate them. It is the task – and the glory – of psychotherapy to help a man caught in the meshes of neurosis, and thus deprived of the freedom to decide upon his own life, by showing him the way to arrive at a true picture of himself and his place in the order of being, of his task and his hope.

The psychiatrist, even though he may be a religious man, does not have the task of preaching good tidings; but to him it is given to "prepare the ways of the Lord and make straight His paths."

REFLECTIONS ON CO-OPERATION AND COMMUNICATION

It would be an abuse of your time, and mine, were I to explain at length how greatly I feel honored and how deeply I am moved by the award lust conferred on me. And even if I were to make such an attempt, I would hardly know what words to chose. The expression of my profound gratitude is also due to the Most Rev. Bishop of Jefferson City for his all too kind citation. I have to admit, however, that I am not a little embarrassed by seeing me, as it were, anatomized in public. The more so, since the Thomas Aquinas Medal has not been awarded to me because I happen to be this person and having this history, but for what I may have achieved as a scholar and as a teacher.

The biography of a scholar is, in most cases, not particularly interesting; it does not furnish the material out of which is made what newspaper people call a "human interest story," which for that matter may tell much of what is human but little of what is of interest. A scholar disappears behind his work; only what he has done counts. Only few of those engaged in scholarly activities may hope that their work will last or be known to future generations, and how much of it will be of permanent significance the author himself does not know. One has to be a poet, and therefore something of a prophet, to claim with Horace *Exegi monumentum aere perennius*. But' the contributions of those whose names and writings have been forgotten and are remembered only when a candidate looks for a topic on which to write his dissertation or because they were fortunate enough to have had among their pupils a real great man, even those humble collaborators in the unending task of scholarly endeavor have not labored in vain. For each of them co operates, in an however modest degree, in this unending task and is, if nothing other, a link between those who went before and those still to come. Communication, indeed, exists not only between contemporaries; it is perfectly meaningful to say that Plato or Aristotle, Thomas or Rant "speak to us" to day as they spoke to so many generations and will speak to many more.

It is in consequence of considerations of this kind that I propose to talk to you on certain "Reflections on Co-operation and Communication."

The problems falling under these titles have been present at all times. But they have come to the fore with a particular urgency in these our days. We are witnessing, as is generally known, a shrinking of our planet; distance disappears; isolation is no longer possible. What happens to individuals or to nations depends on the intricate network of global relations. The time is past in which a man or a people could remain indifferent to what went on in some distant part of the globe.

Accordingly, Norbert Wiener distinguishes three main periods of technological endeavor; the first period is characterized by the tendency to diminish the amount of human effort; the second by the measures aiming at the best possible utilization of energy; the third by the development of means of communication. This term must be understood in a wide sense so as to comprise not only transmission of verbal messages but also transportation of material things. The importance of the last named aspect is easily realized when one considers the decentralization of industrial production, that is the fact that parts of a complex product are made in often very distant places, and also by the need of importing raw materials from far off countries.

But communication is seen in such considerations exclusively as taking place in the present. One all too easily forgets that the present is significant only by virtue of its containing and continuing the past. Without the past's " speaking to the living" the present would be meaningless. And it is the study of the communication coming to us from the past which may serve best for an elucidation of the nature of communication. Such a study involves two problems which, without being independent of each other, are sufficiently distinct to allow separate treatment. There is, first, the problem, or the set of problems, which may be comprised under the heading of a phenomenology of communication. We know by far not enough about the characteristics of the several communicative situations, means of communication, conditions of efficacy, and so on, in spite of the analysis worked out by Husserl and his emphasis on intersubjectivity and in spite also of the contributions made by analytic philosophy and semantics. Of this problem, however, I do not • intend to talk.

The second problem may be designated as that of an ontology of communication. One has to ask: What makes communication possible? What is the ontological status of that which is communicated? What place holds within the framework of an encompassing ontology what we call "meaning?"

Similar questions have to be asked in regard to co operation, and even more fundamentally in regard to "operation", that is, to man's creativity, the production of works, and so on.

These are, I submit, very important questions to which one has not, perhaps, given all the attention they deserve. Some of these questions have arisen in the context of contemporary, so-called "existentialistic" philosophies. When Heidegger speaks of being with, *Mitsein*, as a constitutive aspect of the human situation, or J. P. Sartre makes similar statements, though with a very different slant, or Gabriel Marcel stresses *être-avec* and *communion*, they imply, of course, that one has to do not simply with a statement on human nature or man's situation, but also with a datum of human experience. But none of these thinkers asks, so far as I know, what renders this experience possible. And when the students of semantics or of analytic philosophy inquiry into the meaning of words they likewise presuppose that this meaning may be conveyed from a sender to a recipient without, however, inquiring into the ontological conditions which make this transmission of meaning possible.

Antecedent to all such questions one has to ask another. It is clear that communication, and subsequently co operation, is an intersubjective event. We do not communicate in the strict sense of the term with any non human being; if we flatter ourselves that we do, it is by means of an imaginative transforming an animal into a quasi person. And it is only by means of a more or less sentimental metaphor that one may speak of " communing with nature." Hence, the presupposition of all communication is that the one to whom we address ourselves be recognized as our like. Now, the question of how we know that a certain thing within our environment is a human is not one to be answered by psychology, or at least, not only by psychology. It may be that the question cannot be answered because one has to do with a fundamental trait of human nature. But before we decide to resign ourselves to a simple acceptance of the fact, we have to try all we may possibly do to find a satisfactory solution.

But this is neither a matter on which I want to talk, the more so, since to discuss it much more time would be needed than I have at my disposal. But it seemed advisable to mention these topics, be it only in passing, to show how far the problematics extend which appear before us, once we approach the facts of communication within the framework of ontological reasoning. It may also be that by doing so we become aware of vistas of which we have been almost ignorant up to now.

The central problem related to communication is, I believe, that of the ontological status of the matter which is communicated. Only when we can achieve clarity on this point will it be possible to inquire into the nature of the relation between the means of communication and that to which they refer or that which they are to convey.

I have remarked that communication exists not only among contemporaries but also among our predecessors and ourselves. The fact that the past "speaks to us" may even be particularly revealing. The past speaks in many ways, but obviously most intelligibly when the words spoken and put down centuries ago have been preserved and deciphered. Here the problem becomes most obvious: what sort of ontological status can be attributed to the "message"? What the inscription newly excavated, the papyrus deciphered have to say was there, indeed, all the time; but it cannot be said to have existed, although it persisted. But this it did because the material thing, the stone or the paper were not destroyed; they were and are existent realities. But what they mean cannot be said to be "real" in the same sense.

In such cases the meaning or message remains hidden; it persists unimpaired through many centuries. In fact, however, this is something that happens continually in the communicative situation and appears only magnified, as it were, in the case of the deciphered inscription. Any message east in a code is mute for someone who cannot decode the text, as the hieroglyphs were mute before Champollion found the key. But mute or not, the message is "there" and the manner in which it is there, in its material setting, is a problem of ontology. It is in fact, *the* problem to be studied if one wants to arrive at an understanding of the phenomena which constitute the universal human fact of communication.

For the same relation between the message and its material support or setting exists whenever people communicate with each other. A letter is an instance of the same phenomenon one observes in the case of the unearthed inscription; while the letter travels from the writer to the addressee the message remains bidden, inactive, but again it is "there." A letter takes hours or days to reach its destination; only a fraction of a second elapses between the utterance of a speaker and the understanding of the listener. But one easily sees that the situation is the same.

Be the time long or short that passes from the moment the message became enshrouded in the material phenomena which convey it, there is always a time during which the message has a peculiar mode of being. Peculiarity does not say much; one must try to characterize this mode of being more precisely. This I believe to be feasible, first, by indicating certain features which can be stated in an affirmative manner, and secondly, by pointing out, negatively, what differences there are between this mode of being and others which ontology recognizes.

What strikes one first is, no doubt, that one has to do with "dependent being." The message requires a physical medium in which it is enshrined and by which it is supported and conveyed. Whether there may be also a non material support is a question to he taken up later. In any case, the message has its being only insofar as it is supported. I have suggested, on previous occasions, that this mode of being might appropriately be designated as that of "insistence."

A short time ago I referred to the fact that "insistent being" does not exist as a reality. What exists is the supporting medium: But insistent being, on the other band, shares with existing being the power of efficiency. In fact, there is no other power as effective as that of insistent being on the level of rationality and human co existence. All what renders intersubjective relations possible rests on the efficacy of messages; information, persuasion, command, questioning, all ways of coming to a mutual understanding, hence also all co-operation are founded, at least in an overwhelming majority of cases, on actual, present or on antecedent transmission of a message. It is certainly not the physical form in which the message is transmitted which re leases a response on the part of the recipient. One and the same message may be conveyed by very different supporting media; this is sufficiently evidenced by the fact that one and the same message can be conveyed in very different manners, different words, different languages, orally or by writing, and so on. The message becomes effective only when it is "understood," that is, when it is, if one may say so, "taken out" by the recipient of its material support. The sounds we hear, the letters we read, have as such no power; they neither convince us nor do they make us act.

One has to realize, however, that not much is said by simply referring to "understanding." A more detailed examination of this operation will reveal that there are several operations falling under this title. One understands a word when one knows its meaning as stated in a dictionary. But every word is surrounded by a halo of connotations, different in each language and also within the same language according to the particular universe of discourse in which the word appears. This higher level of understanding may be called the apprehension of the "concrete concept" in the sense in which Hegel uses this term. Understanding a context is again another operation and may re quire what is commonly called "interpretation." I cannot here elaborate on these matters which, however, appear to me as of paramount importance for a philosophy of communication and, hence, of all kinds of "being with."

I beg to avail myself of this opportunity for coming back to a remark I made in the discussion on existentialism at the last meeting of this Association. I then qualified the etymological and interpretative acrobatics in which Mr. Heidegger indulges as "tricks." Someone, more charitable than I ever can hope to be, suggested that one replace the term "trick" by that of "technique." Well, all right: technique. But I would like to remind you that there are also the techniques of pick pockets and magicians, and very effective techniques they are.

Insistent being, therefore, is endowed with efficacy and nevertheless not real.

These two features, dependency and efficacy, are, I submit, perfectly obvious. They are also, for the moment, all that may be said of insistent being in an affirmative way. Other characteristics can be discovered only by comparing the mode of insistence with other modes of being, hence, negatively.

Insistent being evidently is *esse in alio*; But is it the same *esse in* as that proper to accidents? At fist sight it seems that it is. That the message is intelligible only under certain conditions is not an objection against its being viewed as an accident; there are accidents which become manifest only by virtue of some situation, as e.g. magnetism to be manifest requires the presence of a piece of iron. But an accident needs a substance in which to inhere. And it is hardly possible to attribute substantiality to a word, a sentence, or to whatever support a message may have. Here arises another problem which, I believe, has not as yet been sufficiently investigated: that of the ontological status of the means of communication. Though this is not the place for any further discussion of this problem, I might point out, nevertheless, its significance by referring to the fact that not only single words or sentences but whole contorts of the latter convey a definite message. A poem, for instance, is certainly a whole and the message it conveys is supported not by the individual words but by this whole. And it is the message Which confers wholeness on the poem. While all this is rather obvious, the nature or the ontological status of both message and poem remain obscure. But if this point cannot be clarified an appraisal of "analytic philosophy" or the "analysis of language" will lack foundation.

Since that wherein the message insists cannot well be considered as a substance, it is neither possible to envisage the message as an accident. But both, message and accident, are *entia in alio*. Consequently, it would deem that this term *esse in alio* is not as unequivocal as it is generally assumed.

The insistent being insists in its support but becomes manifest only if and when the message is understood or appears as meaningful to some recipient. As long as this is not the case the message remains latent. But this latency must not be identified with *esse in potentia*. For nothing is actualized in the supporting being by the act of understanding. Buried and unread, the inscription is the same as it is after it has been excavated and deciphered. An actualization, indeed, takes place; but in the mind of the recipient. Which is another way to say that insistent being is effective without being real or existent.

Actualization, however, presupposes some *esse in actu*. But can insistent being be said to be in act? It has to be, for otherwise it could not convey anything to the mind of the recipient and thus become "information" in the strict sense of the term. Since the message "informs," the question arises whether or in what sense the message may be considered as of the nature of a form.

Undoubtedly, it shares with the form the property of being able to become detached from something and to pass over into something other as it happens in all kinds of cognition (in other instances, too, which need not concern us). The message passes from the mind of the sender into the physical medium of communication and from there into the mind of the recipient. Communication is essentially imparting of information. For the sharp division many to day make between factual and emotive utterances is, I dare say, rather artificial. Every utterance is at once presentation, appeal and expression. Understanding a message means under all circumstances receiving some sort of information.

As soon, however, as one tries to argue on the basis of this apparent similarity of formal and insistent being one encounters insurmountable difficulties. Of what could the message possibly be the form? If it is feasible, though not without doing some violence to the notion, to consider the message as a form, accidental form, of the mind either of the sender or of the recipient, it is not possible to view in the same manner the relation of the message and its material support. Furthermore, there is the fact that one and the same message may be conveyed by very different media, stated in this language or that other one, transmitted by acoustical or electric waves, put down in writing or recorded on a tape. One must not be misled by the use of the term "form" in regard to works of literature or art. There is certainly some similarity of this meaning of "form" or also "structure" and the notion of form as used in ontology. But the differences are equally evident and, I believe, greater, than any similarities. In innumerable instances such similarities are not found at all; a message may be conveyed by a single word or a single gesture in which ease one cannot speak of structure or anything resembling the "form" of a poem or an essay.

That what constitutes the "meaning" of a word, a sentence, a treatise, or to use an expression I have suggested previously – the verbal, propositional and contextual referents, cannot be viewed as form or as something akin to form. Nor can the mental operation by the means of which the recipient becomes cognizant of the message be said to be of the same kind as that of "abstraction." We neither abstract meaning in general, nor the particular message conveyed in a single instance. "Understanding" a sentence or a speech is something other than apprehending the nature of a substantial being. One has to do with an intellectual operation of which animals, no doubt, are incapable; they do not truly "understand" words, but respond to them, by virtue of appropriate training, as acoustical signals, that is, as concrete elements of a concrete, actual situation. But the operation commonly called understanding cannot be subsumed wader any of the types of intellectual operations we enumerate in psychology, empirical or philosophical.

Notwithstanding the peculiar nature of understanding and of what is understood, that is the message or the insistent being, there is something characteristic of a message which makes it resemble form. Namely, its timelessness. As the being of forms is independent of their being actualized in an existent, so that of insistent being is not affected by its being incorporated in a material support, by its being or not being understood, or by its being encountered by a potential recipient. We do not and cannot know what the message was the lost parts of a philosophical work, say, of Heraclitus, did convey; but this is only because the material support has been lost, not because the message itself perished. Once a message has been, as it were, horn it may persist for ever. Nor is it ever "replaced" by another. If I have come to realize that an opinion I believed to be true has been disproved, I withdraw my consent to it; but the message, now labelled erroneous, does not vanish. It persists in the mode of negation. If I say: previously I thought this, but now I know that I have to think that, the false notion stays with me; otherwise I could not make such a statement. Were it not so that the message is exempt of all destruction, one could not speak of a "history of ideas."

It would be interesting to inquire into the significance the tacitly recognized timelessness of the message played in certain philosophical conceptions. It is not impossible that this feature, together with the peculiar efficacy proper to the message to some extent determined Plato to ascribe reality, even of the highest order, to the "ideas." But it is not here the place to pursue any further this line of thought.

From all I have said hitherto, however incomplete and sketchy it be, follows, or so it seems to me, that "insistent being" constitutes an ontological region *sui generis*. And that it is by virtue of this " participation" in this ontological region that human individuals can communicate with each other and, therefore, also co operate in a common enterprise. Mere rationality of human nature and the ability to speak are not enough to render communication and co operation possible.

Human beings encounter each other, run into each other, are welcome or a nuisance to each other in the world of things, of space and of time. But as minds and, therefore, as persons they meet in the realm of insistent being.

For this realm extends farther than the foregoing remarks 1mplied. First, it is obviously the same mode of being that is proper to the message when it has become incorporated in a conveying support and when it is still present only in the mind of the sender or apprehended and understood by the mind of the recipient. Intentional being or the mode of being belonging to the intentional object is, I submit, the same as that of the message insistent in its support. Prior to the invention of script there was no other way for insistent being to persist than its retention in the mind of an individual. Seen from the angle of ontology there is no essential difference between oral and scriptural tradition. And the "messenger" who originally conveyed a message from one person to another was not the written word but the message was entrusted to a person who acted as mediator between a sender and a recipient. And it is still so in innumerable instances to day.

Secondly, human understanding apprehends not only messages properly so called but also situations. Not only persons but things, too, "speak to us." A situation is meaningful to one and void of meaning to another. One understands it and the other fails to do so. To one a given situation presents a challenge while another remains unaffected. The relation, then, between a person and the situation by which he is faced, is not unlike that between him and the message which reaches him end which he either understands or fails to recognize as what it is.

It is with good reason that language knows of the expression "understanding a situation," that is, realizing what demands it makes on one, and acting in accord with these demands. A situation, indeed, becomes humanly relevant inasmuch as it is "understood." One might say, without expanding unduly the meaning of the term, that a situation, when understood, has a message for us. This message takes on several forms which to describe is a task of philosophical anthropology, not to be undertaken now. It is not enough simply to say that it pertains to man's nature that he be in a world; the several modes of this being in as also those of being with have to be distinguished and characterized.

Being in a world and being with others is mediated through the message insisting in all sorts of situations, be they those of communication by words and their substitutes or those requiring action, individual or concerted. Insistent being is the one and only means by which human relations as well as the relations of man to his environment come to be established. It seems to me that the failure to recognize this all important rôle of insistent being underlies the claim of contemporary "existentialist" philosophy to have "abolished" the cleavage between subject and object, a cleavage which, according to the words of one author, "has bedevilled the human mind since the beginning of the modem age." The reference is, obviously, to the Cartesian doctrine of the two substances, the *res extensae* and the *res cogitantes*. This doctrine has, as one knows, become a stumbling block to philosophical speculation, especially in regard to the mind-body relation and the problem of epistemology. This needs no further illustration. But it may be pointed out that one of the difficulties arising from the position of Descartes is the impossibility of there being any trait common to the two substances. As long as the sharp distinction of the two substances is maintained, there is, indeed, no way to arrive at an understanding of the unity of the human person and the interaction of mind and body on one hand, and of the mind's reaching out into the surrounding world and knowing or transforming it on the other hand. The notion of the one substance with the attributes of spirit and matter in Spinoza, the appeal to God as mediator in occasionalism, the idea of pre established harmony of Leibniz, to some extent also Kant's philosophy, they all aim at overcoming this difficulty.

Now, no one will deny that there is a profound difference between mind and matter, and that their interaction requires an explanation. Nor that an ontological foundation must be assumed for all intersubjectivity. But it seems impossible to find a way out of the subject, to conceive of him otherwise than as enclosed in himself, as long as one places oneself on the stand point of the pure *cogito*. This has been recognized, for instance, by Leibniz who pointed out that the mere *cogito* does not allow for an explanation of the diversity of the *cogitationes* and that, therefore, account must be taken of the *cogitata* as independent of, and given to, the subject. M. Gilson has not long ago emphasized the impossibility to arrive at a metaphysics of given reality when the *cogito* is chosen as the starting point. Particularly, it is the fact of intersubjectivity, of communication and co-operation, which remains inexplicable if envisaged from the Cartesian standpoint. Husserl was keenly aware of the necessity to find an ontological basis for intersubjectivity and also for the totality of the immediately given, the "lived world," *Lebenswelt*; but it does not seem that he has been able to transcend the walls Descartes has built around the solitary *ego cogitans*. Notwithstanding all the efforts Husserl made there is, so far as I can see, no means to pass over from the transcendental consciousness which "constitutes" all that is given in a trans subjective reality which would be, if one may say so, self-supporting.

Nor can I see that the existentialists have been able really to bridge the gap between subject and object. In fact, one does not find in their writings much more than the mere affirmation that this feat has been achieved. I confess that this affirmation is to me unintelligible. It does not convey any message with the exception of that it reveals the problem blindness with which these thinkers are not less afflicted than many others. As odor blindness so problem blindness exists in several forms; the positivist, the naturalist, the materialist, the existentialist suffer each of their own kind of problem blindness. That the subject be set over against an object, that the ego knows himself as distinct from all that constitutes the non ego, that all consciousness as Husserl himself emphasized is of something other than itself these are primordial facts which cannot he explained away

A critical analysis of existentialism would have to raise the question why this so called bridging of the gap between subject and object appears to these thinkers as an important advance over the philosophical conceptions hitherto accepted. Although this inquiry is beyond the scope of my talk, I would like to point out that there are apparently several reasons. There i, first, the belief that all metaphysics has to start somehow from the Cartesian standpoint, and that the one conception which may be said to bridge this gap, namely Hegelian idealism, is unacceptable. Secondly, there is the claim of naturalism and materialism to have closed the gap by viewing the subject as part or element of nature, so that subjectivity would no longer appear as a feature by which the world of the given is split into two parts. A similar influence is exercised by Marxism which has penetrated also minds which want to be anything but Marxists. Thirdly, there is the fact that many of the contemporary thinkers and not only the existentialists harbor an all too narrow conception of "object." They seem to believe Gabriel Marcel for instance that "object" must be defined in terms of science, therefore, as something which does not concern the person qua person and is, in fact, independent of individual experience because, being "objectively true," it is exactly the same for all persons. What is overlooked in such arguments is that "object" is not an univocal term. All that is apprehended by the subject as pertaining to the non ego is "object", is "set over against," whatever the nature of the apprehending act may be intuition, love, awareness of mystery, or what not.

I venture to submit that the problem of the subject object relation takes on a different aspect if the mediating rôle of insistent being is recognized. For this being, as I tried to make clear, is indifferent in regard to the nature of its support. It is the same as insistent in the mind as the intentional object and as constituting the meaning or message of an utterance or any other creation of the human mind. Because it is neither an *esse existentiae* nor an *esse essentiae* but *sui generis* it may be seen as bridging the gap between subject and object, not by abolishing it but by mediating between two worlds.

It furthermore seems to me that the recognition of this mode of being may well enable us to construct an ontology of civilization or to outline a metaphysics of culture. For civilization consists in the gradual transformation of the given raw material of experience into meaningful artifacts. The ontology of the artifact, however, has always been a moot question. A metaphysics of civilization or a philosophy of culture has to take account of the phenomena of development and continuity. Culture and its advance are rendered possible by the communication of the past with the present. One may even say that there is also a cc operation of the present with the past inasmuch as we continue and sometimes complete the work initiated by our ancestors.

In a poem by the Swiss poet Conrad Ferdinand Meyer, *Der Chor der Toten*, the dead speak to the living:

> Und was wir an gültigen Sätzen gefunden,
> Dran bleibt aller irdisclier Wandel gebunden.

The truths we, your predecessors, have found go on determining all human affairs. They that went before are no more. What exists in this sublunar world is bound to vanish. But man has been endowed by his Creator with the power of creativity, not indeed, to bring forth existence but to transform that which merely exists into a meaningful world. It is man's prerogative that he may, by inserting messages into the world that is merely there, by incorporating what insists but lacks existence into the material world bring forth what without him would not be at all: the whole world of artifacts, of products, institutions, interpretations, in one word the world of culture which is that in which man truly lives and moves and has his being.

The realm of insistent being is timeless, and as such not a moving image of eternity, as Plato said of time, but a stable one. Not that it were exempt of change; but this change is not that of coming and ceasing to be; it is the succession of being believed to be true and recognized to be false. But what to day is recognized as an error still persists, though in the form of negation. And as such it is far from having lost all significance; not only does the error of the past serve as a warning to the present at least, it should, even if man does not always heed the voices of the past , it also happens that what one generation discarded as obsolete re emerges in the next generation and takes on a new significance. That the history of ideas knows of what may be termed the "neo-phenomena" neo-Platonism, neo-Classicism, neo-Thomism, and so on finds its explanation in the timelessness of insistent being.

It is part of the unique position bestowed on man by his Creator that he, man, be entrusted not only with the preservation but also with the transformation of this sublunar world.

This is, I take it, the meaning or one of the meanings of the words that have been said of man:

Gloria et honore coronasti eum, Et posuisti eàm super opera manuuns Tuarum.

ONTOANALYSIS:
A NEW TREND IN PSYCHIATRY

Some years ago, certain ideas which had become current in European psychiatry began to gain influence on American psychiatry. There have existed for a couple of years two groups which have assimilated these ideas. The Association of Existential Psychology and Psychiatry edited last year the mimeographed *Existential Inquiries* which grew into the *Review of Existential Psychology and Psychiatry*, the first issue being published in the winter of 1961. The other group calls itself the Ontoanalytic Society and has published since the spring of 1960 the *Journal of Existential Psychiatry*. I have been unable to discover what differences there are between the two groups nor to find any statement that would define their respective aims. I shall, therefore, use the terms "ontoanalysis" and "existential psychiatry" as interchangeable ... especially since such terms as *Daseinsanalyse, existential analyse, psychanalyse existentielle*" and others, which originated in Europe around 1930, have become part of the vocabulary of continental psychiatry.

These names reveal the fact that *psychiatry has felt the need to turn for guidance and inspiration to the new philosophies which are comprised, with more or less justification, under the general title existentialism.* As the use of the term *Dasein* indicates, it is primarily the philosophy of *Martin Heidegger* which has appealed to the psychiatrists – not the whole of this philosophy, however, as it was developed in Heidegger's later works, but those parts which are contained in the writings *prior to 1930*, that is, *Sein und Zeit*, published in 1927, the lecture *Was it Metaphysik?* of 1929 and, to some extent, the essay *Vom Wesen des Grundes*, also of 1929. And of these works, too, only certain parts became significant for psychiatry, namely, those that deal with "*Philosophical anthropology.*" Now, it is known that Heidegger's concern is not primarily with the Dasein, that is, the human being, but with Being as such, and that the "fundamental analysis of the *Dasein*" is undertaken with the intention of finding a way of approach to the *Seinsfrage*, the question of being. It is not for this brief report to ask whether or not this limitation to a particular and preparatory part of the philosopher's ideas entails a certain misinterpretation, nor does time permit to inquire into the reasons why it is just Heidegger's philosophy which appeared as relevant to the psychiatrists.

Philosophy, on the whole, is not accustomed to see her ideas utilized by empirical disciplines. Even less is she disposed to lay down rules or to propose viewpoints of which the empiricist ought to take account. Such attempts have been made twice, once, at the time of the Renaissance and the birth of modern science, and again by German Idealism, especially by Schelling and his followers. Both these attempts ended with a defeat of philosophy. *It is astonishing, therefore, to see rise a movement within psychiatry, an empirical discipline, which openly declares its allegiance to and dependence upon a definite philosophy.*

But the fact remains; and it poses several questions. We have time to consider only a few of these. We may disregard, obviously, all questions of a specifically psychiatric nature, as, for instance, that of the significance of the "existential approach" for diagnosis and treatment or that of its relation to other aspects of psychiatric endeavor. *But we have to ask what particular features of the psychiatrist's work and problem have brought about this turning to philosophy.* In trying to answer this question we shall, at the same time, learn whether in this new relation philosophy is only the giving part or whether she is not, as it were, *somehow repaid for the assistance she lends to psychiatry. I hope to show that the latter is, indeed, the case.*

If there is any trait common to the several forms of existentialism, it is the concern with the human individual in his uniqueness. This concern is also that of the psychiatrist in his dealing with his client. The problem of grasping or understanding the individual, however, takes on a particularly poignant form in the psychotherapeutic situation. Therapy, of course, demands that the psychiatrist avail himself of his knowledge of human nature and of its deviations for the sake of helping the clients return to normalcy. In the psychotherapeutic situation, therefore, there arises a dilemma; or in other words, it is essential to this situation that it have a dialectical structure. For, on the one hand, the psychiatrist has to make use of his general, scientific knowledge, and on the other hand, to deal with an individual who, in his individuality, escapes all attempts at being defined or comprised by any such generality. In fact, the psychotherapeutic situation reveals on an enlarged scale the essential problematic of all medical activity. For it is the task of medicine to apply the data furnished by medical science to the individual "case." But the patient, as an individual and as this one sick individual is not an impersonal "case" that would "fall under" some general laws designated by the diagnosis. The "history," as it appears in medical publications loses its sense and is replaced by the "history of a sick person." (The difference can be expressed more sharply in German where one may oppose, as I did in 1925, the *Krankengeschichte* to the *Geschichte eines Kranken.*) One may go further and say that this same dialectics becomes evident whenever we are faced with the task of applying our scientific and theoretical knowledge of human nature and human conduct in an individual instance, for example, in the field of education, counselling, appraising the aptitudes for this or that kind of work, and so on.

Once this is realized, it becomes clear also that the same dilemma or dialectics characterizes all truly interpersonal relations. For, whenever we try to understand, to convince, to persuade, or in any way to influence another, we rely, consciously or not, on some general ideas of human nature. It is as if we were saying to ourselves: since he is such and such a person, this rather than another argument will be more appealing to him, or: his reacting in this or that manner is indicative of his being a certain type of person rather than another type. But we can never be perfectly certain because the individual cannot be exhaustively characterized by even a very great number of general features. The most complete inventory of human traits proves insufficient to grasp fully an individual person in his very individuality and uniqueness.

One might argue that no individual can ever be known fully by means of general knowledge. Knowledge, especially scientific knowledge, deals, as Aristotle emphasized, with generalities, and no combination of general statements measures up to these features which constitute individuality. In our practical dealing with the things that surround us, however, this inadequacy of knowledge becomes only seldom a handicap. For, we look at and make use of most things only in one respect; there, are innumerable qualitative notes that can be disregarded. These notes, proper to an individual thing, moreover, become more and more insignificant the lower the level of being is to which the individual thing belongs. The thing remains, of course, an individual, but the significance it has for us depends much more on its specific than on its individual nature. The insignificance of the individualizing notes on the lower levels of being becomes manifest by the fact that one thing may replace perfectly another thing of the same kind. This is sufficiently evident to render superfluous any further illustrations.

All that has been said up to this point is rather obvious. It has to be admitted, however, that philosophy – under the influence of the Greek conception of *theoría* as superior to *praxis* – has been relatively neglectful of the problems arising in practical, especially in interpersonal situations. Consequently, it has almost completely been overlooked that the term "individual" is not univocal, but *analogical*. To be an individual does not have the same meaning on the several levels of being.

The relative insignificance of the individualizing notes on the lower existential levels makes it possible that beings belonging to these orders replace each other, regardless of their individuality. On the higher levels, however, such a replacement of one individual by another becomes possible only, when the individual is first subjected to a deindividualizing process which is done most effectively by viewing him as not more than an element in an "organization"; for one has to remember that in "organization" there is no reference to an organism but only *to órganon* in the original sense of "implement."

It is against this de individualization that such existential thinkers as Martin Buber and Gabriel Marcel turn. And it is also that which ontoanalysis seeks to overcome in viewing the person strictly as a unique individual. This entails, furthermore, that the client of the existential analyst be envisaged in the totality not only of his being but also of the circumstances of his life or of his "situation." In this respect Heidegger's statement that to be in a world is constitutive, for the *Dasein*, or in his terminology an *existentiale*, attained a particular importance for the psychiatrist. Envisaged from this angle, the person and his world or his situation form an indissoluble unity. Consequently, the dismemberment of this whole into relatively independent elements, which is the basic procedure of science and of discursive reasoning, is considered to be inadequate. Discursive reasoning, even though indispensable as a tool, does not yield a real insight into an individual; rather, to understand and therefore, to help a person one has to start from "intuition" and to return to it. Since "intuition" is a highly ambiguous term and, especially, often believed to be of an emotional nature, I prefer to speak of a "global apprehension." And I would like to note in passing that the phenomenology of the varieties of global apprehension has still to be worked out; they range from the apprehension of a configuration (*Gestalt*) to that of the individuality of a human person, from that of the apprehension of a simple geometrical order to that of a work of art, so that here, too, we have to do with an analogical term. This has to be realized in order to escape the confusion – to which some students of psychology have fallen prey – which arises when all objects of global apprehension are comprised under the general title of *Gestalt*. The over all characteristic of the objects of global apprehension may be designated as that of a "structured whole;" this term seems to apply to such data as a landscape, a picture, a situation, as well as to what I have once described as the "contextual referent" of a paragraph, a speech, a book or a system.

Whether or not one agrees with the notion just outlined, it will be obvious to most students of this question that it deals with the relation of a mental performance and its trans subjective correlate, that is, its object. Not so with the existential psychiatrists. For one need not read long in the literature dealing with existential psychiatry or ontoanalysis before coming upon the statement that one of the great achievements of the new philosophies consists in having "bridged the gap between subject and object" or "abolished the opposition of subject and object" or, in the words of one of these authors, to have "cut below the cleavage between subject and object which has bedeviled Western thought and science since shortly after the Renaissance." In fact, this claim of having done away with the subject object opposition is usually accompanied by a reference to Descartes as to the one who introduced or, at least, brought to the fore this opposition.

Those who make this claim think primarily of the conditions determining our understanding of another person; they hold that the other person cannot be viewed as an "object" without missing his essential nature as a person. But the mention of science in the sentence just quoted and other similar remarks show that this so called "undercutting" is meant in a general sense. This becomes clear also by the reference, frequently made, to the statement of Heisenberg that scientific data can no longer be considered as objective, but that the experience of nu clear physics forces us to admit the intrusion of a "subjective" element into our apparently "objective" equations.

It is easy to see that in such statements there is a confusion of two meanings of the term " objective." In one sense, this term designates a datum which is the same for all recipients and has to be accepted by all because it corresponds to reality it self, independently of the person who avers it. This is what is meant by the "objectivity of science."

In another sense, how ever, object designates any datum whatsoever inasmuch as it is the referent of some mental act. All consciousness, said Husserl, is consciousness of something, and that of which we are conscious is the object with which we are concerned. To avoid this confusion I prefer to speak of the totality of all referents, correlated to mental acts, as the realm of the "trans subjective." For not only the things apprehended by our senses, but also the "state of affairs" expressed or expressible in a proposition, the goal we desire to attain, the situation which releases an emotional response are "transsubjective; "they are "intentional objects." No matter to what extent something "outside the mind" may be modified or even distorted by the mode of the subjective, apprehending act, this something does not cease to be the "other" of this act. Thus, when the physicist says that his own doing, the means he uses to study, measure and describe a physical phenomenon, disturb this phenomenon and that we never can get hold of facts as they are when we do not interfere with them, the phenomenon, nevertheless, does not cease to be "trans-subjective."

This admixture of a subjective element is said to render meaningless the old conception of objectivity; even the supposedly objective statements of science show themselves to be subjective; what was believed to be a description of reality as independent of the observer appears now as colored, so to speak, by man's doings and the peculiarities or limitations of his being. To keep separate the objective and the subjective is no longer possible.

In truth, however, these discoveries of modern science do not lend any support to the claim that the gap between object and subject has been bridged. For this conclusion rests on a confusion of the two meanings of objectivity I referred to. It is objectively true that there enters into the statements of science, under certain conditions, a subjective factor. This can be verified; it can be observed by an indeterminate number of observers; and a statement on probability, because of the admixture of a subjective element, is not less "trans subjective" than one which does not take account of this admixture, which appears as a feature of the data observed and not as one pertaining to the realm of subjective experience. Without elaborating on this point, I would like to submit that one ought to distinguish between the objectivity and the reliability of a statement or measurement. And one might add that this emphasis on the subjective element does, after all, not say much more than what is contained in the age old principle that *omnia recipiuntur secundum modum recipientis.*

What the mind apprehends does not become subjective by the mere fact that the mode of apprehension is not that believed to be proper to science. Global apprehension, as I called it, does not lend itself to the kind of dismemberment which makes up the essence of the scientific method. This fact, however, can be used as an argument against the cleavage between subject and object only if objectivity is first defined in the manner of scientism and positivism. It should not be forgotten that one may make objectively valid statements on subjective data.

The lack of semantic clarity, so it seems to me, is mainly what makes possible the claim that the opposition of subject and object has been eliminated. There are also other factors at work which deserve discussion, were there enough time. One of these factors may be characterized as a sort of sentimental self deception which leads a person to believe in a peculiar oneness with another person or even with a work of art. The expression "losing oneself" in another person, a painting, or a work of music, shows how strong the temptation is to indulge in this belief. This leads furthermore to a misinterpretation of the togetherness of the We which is taken to be a substantial union. This is a misinterpretation because therein is overlooked the fact that nothing can abolish the otherness of the other. (It must be noted that this is recognized by some of the existentialist psychiatrists.) Whether it be possible to say that we may achieve, under particular conditions, a direct contact, so to speak, with the existential or substantial being of another, is a question requiring careful and penetrating investigation. Even if the answer were in the affirmative, the basic fact of the otherness of the other would not disappear.

Accepting the thesis of ontoanalysis as it apparently is meant would be tantamount to attributing to the We – as well as to other experienced forms of togetherness – an ontological or existential status of its own. Or, in other words, one would have to assume that there exists a new substantial something, an idea hardly compatible with the principles of most philosophies. It might find, perhaps, a place within the framework of Hegelian idealism, but even there it would not he a phenomenal datum but only a stage in the process of the self unfolding of the Absolute. The only conception within which this idea appears as legitimate is that of Eastern mysticism as it is expressed, for instance, in the Mésnevi, a great poem of a Persian mystic: "there dies the Ego, the dark despot." How very different sound the words of Meister Eckhardt: "If thou art in loving union with God and hearest thy brother call for help, let God go and help thy brother."

The proponents of ontoanalysis rely, as I remarked, almost exclusively on the philosophical anthropology they find – or believe to find – in the works of Martin Heidegger. But I cannot discover there any statement that would support the claim of ontoanalysis. Heidegger, indeed, speaks of being in the world and of being with as of *existentialia,* as basic traits of the mode of being proper to the *Dasein.* But this does not deprive the world or the fellow man of their ontological status, of their being in their own right. These terms are rather indicative of the self-transcendence of the *Dasein.*

Ontoanalysis might refer, with the semblance of more justification, to certain utterances by Gabriel Marcel who emphatically declares that the Thou can never become an object without being deprived of its very nature. Marcel, however, takes the term "object" exclusively as designating that aspect of reality which is investigated by science. What he means to say is that the scientific, analytic, impersonal approach is inadequate in our relation to each other. (Almost identical statements may be found in the writings of Martin Buber.) In spite of all the emphasis on *communion, engagement* and similar terms, as well as on *le mystère,* with Marcel also, the other retains his being as an ontological entity in himself. This is evidenced, for instance, by two remarks – among – many others – which appeared to Marcel's faithful commentator, Père Troisfontaines, as of so fundamental significance that he uses them as a motto for one part of his treatise; the first reads: ... *le sujet ne se constitue comme sujet qu'à condition de reconnaître l'autre comme étant lui même un sujet,"* that is, the other has to be recognized as likewise a subject and, hence, as an independent being in his own right. The second remark summarizes, in a somewhat paradoxical manner, one of Marcel's basic convictions: *La métaphysique, c'est le prochain.* Marcel views intersubjectivity as a primary datum and as the starting point of metaphysical reflection. Heidegger, on the other hand, starts from the individual Dasein which is always my own – *je meines* – . And thus, he remains, in a way, true to the tradition running from Descartes to Husserl, even though he holds that metaphysics, as it developed since Plato has come to its end with Hegel and Nietzsche. The ideas of Marcel – and also those of Buber – seem to be particularly suitable for a deeper understanding of the problem arising within, and connected with, the psychotherapeutic situation. They have, however, curiously played a relatively subordinate role in the endeavors of the existential psychiatrists to work out the ontological structures underlying the psychotheraputic situation and they have attracted greater attention only in very recent times, when several authors came to realize the basic importance of the "encounter." But stressing this importance seems hardly compatible with the idea of abolishing the opposition of subject and object, if the latter term is correctly understood and not taken as a category peculiar to science.

I have dealt at some length with the question of the subject object relation as it comes to the fore in the encounter of the psychiatrist and his client not because of the emphasis placed on it by the existential psychiatrists and not because of the unacceptability of the answer proposed by them. That some people hold untenable ideas need not he of greater concern to philosophy; she may trust that sooner or later these erroneous ideas will be corrected. But it has to be recognized that, although the solution be insufficient, the problem is a real one and that it has not been studied hitherto as it deserves. In fact, it is not one problem but a whole network of problems which becomes apparent in the psychotherapeutic situation which presents, as I pointed out earlier, aspects common to all truly human encounter on, so to speak, a magnified scale. I have referred to one side of this problem as that of the nature of "global apprehension." I beg to submit some further considerations.

I believe it to be evident that there exists a strict correlation between an intentional act and its object. To every kind of object corresponds a peculiar way of apprehension.

We distinguish the powers of the mind by their objects and their operations. The same principle applies to the several modes in which a power functions. To discover and to characterize these modes is one of the tasks of phenomenology. While for a general philosophy of the mind it suffices that the usual broad distinctions be made, it becomes indispensable for a more detailed study and for a fuller knowledge of human nature that account be taken of further differentiations. These may be such as to cut across, so to speak, the division of the mental powers. Global apprehension, as I have called it, is a peculiar modification of sensory as well as of intellectual awareness. The corresponding objects may be said to possess a structure or to form a context. Some have thought of doing justice to this fact by using the notion of *Gestalt* or configuration in a very broad sense. Therein lies, as I pointed out, the danger that one overlooks the differences by stressing the similarities, that is, the analogical significance of the term. Although it is true that all structures, contexts, meaningful wholes, or whatever name one may prefer, have something in common and that this something – which perhaps, escapes further analysis – is apprehended by a mental operation *sui generis*, it is true also that in apprehending a geometrical configuration, a painting, the structure of a poem, the meaning of an essay, the general nature of a philosophical system, each case has its own peculiarities. The same is true of the apprehension of a human person, be that apprehension of our own person or of another's. That existential psychology and psychiatry have forcibly pointed out this fact, is a notable service rendered to philosophy. I have thought it advisable to concentrate on the significance these new trends in the empirical study of man have for philosophy and to leave aside the question of their meaning for the theoretical and practical endeavors of the psychiatrist. It falls outside the scope of this short presentation to inquire into the particular problems with which philosophy is faced when she tries to come to terms with these new facts and ideas. And this is, I submit, a task philosophy is not allowed to shun if she is to stay alive. Otherwise, it will be her fate to become petrified, to degenerate into mere formalistic discussion, and to lose the capacity to fill the place which is rightfully hers in the order of knowledge.

WORK AND PLAY

In this paper the Author vindicates the traditional difference between work and play against some modern psychological and educational misconceptions. Work is aimed at producing some change, be it however passing, in reality, whereas play is an end in itself. Correspondingly, the gratification resulting from achievement by work is related to the final effect and can be described as the "pleasure of achievement"; the pleasure arising from playing, however, resides in the play activity itself and is a "functional pleasure," It does not seem therefore advisable to prepare children for work by making it playful as if trying to obliterate the difference between the two kinds of activity. Children will realize the true value of work as they grow in general maturity and in social consciousness (Editor's Note).

Not so long ago people were certain that they knew what it means to play and what it means to work. They may not have been able to define the one or the other, but they knew then to he different. There is a time to play and a time to work, they said, implying that the two activities were incompatible with each other; either you play or you work, but you cannot do both at the same time. Or they declared that work is serious and play is not. When used in this context, the term "serious" does not refer, obviously, to a mood or an attitude; children often are very serious when playing, and so may be adults, for instance at the chess board. The meaning is rather that we have in mind when we say that an action has serious consequences or that a person is seriously ill. We call serious facts or events which produce some effect in reality which play does not.

The essential difference between playing and working consists, indeed, in that the latter is aimed at producing some change, be it however passing, in reality, whereas the former is an end in itself. Correspondingly, the gratification resulting from achievement by work is related to the final effect and can be described as the "pleasure of achievement"; the pleasure arising from playing, however, resides in the play activity itself and is a "functional pleasure," The activity of working ends with the attainment of its goal; the activity of playing may go on indefinitely. Children, it would seem, might never cease to play if there were no interference on the part of the adults or if fatigue did not force them to stop.

The opinion quoted above appears thus as well founded, and to pass from play to work or from work to play seems to amount to a *metabasis eis allo genos*. In fact, parents still think as they did in older time, but they have become doubtful; they do not trust their own ideas, since they have been told by the "scientific psychologists" and the several authorities on education that these ideas are quite wrong and that they must heed what these authorities prescribe arid not trust either commonsense or traditional procedures.

Among other ideas proposed by these experts is also that the sharp distinction of play and work is unjustified. They recognize that playing is an activity natural to the child[1] and they want to exploit it for the sake of introducing gradually the child into the world of work by making working appear as playing and play a means for the acquisition of working habits and of useful knowledge. But it is difficult to uproot commonsense and convictions which remained unquestioned for centuries. There are still many people who doubt whether these procedures are justified.

In an American magazine one saw, in the last months of the year, a cartoon which, in anticipation of the time of Christmas shopping, showed a counter in a department store, bearing the inscription "Educational Toys." The man behind the counter, resembling more a teacher than a salesman, looked severely at his customer, a lady with a little boy. And the caption read: "haven't you anything with which the child could just play?" Underlying is the notion that injustice and violence is done to the child when he is deprived of his natural right just to play.

If a small child were capable, *per impossibile*, of expressing his views on these "educational toys," he might say: "It is exactly like them (the adults) that they try to sneak in their ideas into our world which they do not understand," (Many adults would be very amazed and profoundly shocked, were they to realize what children think of them.) Sometimes a child, at the age of passing from childhood to pre adolescence, is quite aware of his leaving one world to enter another. A girl

1 This essay is concerned only with early childhood, including the first years in school. Later many factors enter into play which cannot be discussed here. The re examination and appraisal requires a separate study. Consequently, no detailed mention will be made of the educational significance of sportive activities.

remarked, on her tenth birthday: "I am very glad to be ten, and I shall be glad to be eleven and twelve; later ... I don't know," Asked why, she said: "Then you can't play anymore," She knew, of course, that older children also play and that even adults do. But she was conscious of the fact that the kind of playing which still was hers and her friends' would cease to exist.

For the playing of early childhood is essentially imaginative. It transforms reality and makes it possible that one and the same thing function in most diverse manners. It needs but a minimum support by real things. To sit astride of a chair, a log, or anything suffices for the little boy to imagine himself riding on horseback; a bundle of rags may become a baby in the eyes of the little girl. It is not so much "playing with" as "playing at," Imagination creates a second world which may be much more attractive than the real world; and within this imaginative world children find and understand each other in a truly astonishing manner. Competition may play a certain role, but often is completely absent;[2] a child may play all by himself or play with another child in co operation rather than in competition, as for instance in the case of two girls playing together with their dolls. Reality, of course, cannot be disregarded all together; it is there and asserts itself. Children take account of reality by imitating it; but their imitation is not "true to life," it is an often far going transformation. Since children lack the power to bring about any change in reality, they replace it by a world of their own.[3]

One may question the wisdom of introducing into this world elements which in fact do not pertain to it. I shall return to this point later. First, however, another aspect of modern conceptions regarding the relations of work and play must be briefly characterized.

From the angle of the child the imaginative transformation of reality appears as an improvement; but the realistically minded adult looks

---

2 Huizinga (*Homo ludens*) sees in the competitive or, as he calls it, *agonal* aspect the very essence and the origin of play. This is going too far because thus one overlooks the purely imaginative play which may be also solitary.

3 One may find a poetic and, if one wants to call it so, an allegorical presentation of the facts alluded to above in a lovely story by E. Th. A. Hoffmann, *Des fremde Kind*. There is also, in this tale, a reference to the consciousness children have, when growing up, of an irretrievable loss; something has gone out of their lives which they feel to have had a charm of its own which they will never recapture. Unless one happens to be a true poet.

at it as at a falsification.[4] He wants the child to become acquainted as soon as possible with the world "as it is," He is afraid that the child would be not sufficiently prepared for life if imagination prevailed over a longer time, although innumerable generations have grown up with fairy tales and all sorts of fantastic stories and nevertheless became quite capable of dealing with reality.[5]

But to play is natural for the child and he cannot be wholly prevented from playing. (Although this has happened sometimes, either because of economic conditions – child labor – or because of a narrow minded and over rigoristic mentality.) And playing is, even with "educational" toys, different from working. Modern psychological and educational theories have viewed the passage from play to work as a difficulty which must be overcome and made as light as possible. Hence, the tendency to make work appear as play; it is by playing, for instance at buying and selling, that the child is supposed to become acquainted with the elements of arithmetic. These theories and their applications are so well known that further examples are unnecessary. It is also well known that these new methods of instruction did not yield the results one expected. Recently, more and more people demand that the child be introduced into the world of work and not made believe that there is no difference between work and play. This has been urged by some educators, but chiefly by parents and the teachers in secondary and higher schools who find that the children are badly prepared for any activity which is work in the true sense of the term.

Bygone times did not think it necessary to provide for a gradual transition from play to work. They knew enough means to make the child work, and some of these means were, indeed, very harsh. Since modern education and child psychology is beset by the fear of "frustration" and of causing a lasting damage to the child's personality, all

4 It is because of this attitude that the terms "play" and "playing" are used so very often in a pejorative sense. The impostor, the hypocrite, the intriguer are "playing a role." Finally, play becomes synonymous with planned deception. Dante, speaking of Michael Scotus (*Inf.* XX, 116): *che veramente / Delle magiche frode seppe il guioco.*

5 This may be one of the reasons why toys of a non educational nature are given quite distorted shapes and appear as caricatures. The same applies to many of the so called comic-strips. The idea seems to be that the world of ply and imagination be made different from the real world and the former's unreality be thus emphasized.

harsh measures had to be discarded and other means to be found to – one would almost say – persuade the child that he work. And one of the most obvious means was to make the transition as smooth as possible.

The need of a gradual transition and the dangers of an abrupt change have been, probably, exaggerated. The acquisition of working habits proceeded in general, without major catastrophes; when entering school the child had some knowledge of what it means to work, he had seen the parents working, had observed older children doing their school work, and he had become accustomed to discipline. But times and the spirit that pervades them have changed, and education must take account of this fact. For children grow up in this atmosphere and are exposed to its influence from the moment onwards when their consciousness awakened. In an overwhelming majority of families the children will get the impression that work is tedious, that man works only because he has to earn a living, that the true life is that of leisure and that one of the main goals is to get paid more and more for doing less and less.

This attitude was brought about by the steadily progressing fragmentation of work which, in turn, is the inevitable consequence of the development of technology. The most important feature of this process is, perhaps, not the monotony of so many forms of work, but the disappearance of the pleasure of achievement. Objectively, of course, work is under all conditions productive of lasting values. And reflection may tell the worker that he contributes to the realization of values. But the concrete experience of achievement is gone. (This point needs obviously, considerable elaboration; in the present context, however, we have to be content with these few remarks). This experience, however, is an essential element of a satisfying existence.

Sooner or later the children discover this peculiar experience. "Mother, look what I have *done*," exclaimed the little son of the Scupins one day and his expression showed clearly the intense pleasure this new fact, the fact of having achieved something, gave him. It has been pointed out that this experience is linked not only to the realization of achievement but also to the recognition that this realization was made possible by using the material in an adequate manner (*materialgerecht*, Ch. Buehler).

Achievement is the experience by virtue of which the regions of play and of work border on each other or even overlap. Modern psychology, and consequently also modern theory of education, have not paid sufficient attention to the fact that there are several kinds of pleasure. The pleasure of satisfaction (seeing a desire fulfilled, a need satisfied, etc.) is not the same as the pleasure of function, observable mostly in the playing activity of the child, and the two again differ from the pleasure of achievement. That the second and the third appear later in life than the first is no reason for "deriving" them from the pleasure of satisfaction. Each kind of pleasure has its own peculiar qualitative traits. It is perfectly conceivable that certain factors become actualized at various stages of individual development; they pre exist, of course, as potentialities from the very beginning of life, but a number of conditions has to be fulfilled for their potencies to be actualized.

The imaginative world of pure play evades the difficulties of reality. But achievement proves to the young mind that it is capable of coping with reality. It is difficult to describe the peculiarities of the several kinds of pleasure. But one may point at the sentiment of "triumph" as characteristic of the experience of achievement. The knowledge that he has been able to subject reality to his will is more important to the child than the, in fact rather problematic, need of "self expression," Play activities, therefore, which culminate in an achievement may justly be considered as bridging the gap between "mere playing" and "really working," On closer inspection, however, this answer reveals itself as a too far going simplification; a further distinction becomes necessary.

We may leave aside the cases in which a man falls to experience a sentiment of triumph in spite of his having achieved something as well as the opposite case of an objectively unfounded sentiment of triumph. These are mere errors of judgment as they occur elsewhere too. They point, however, at the unreliability of the subjective criterion. This unreliability becomes even more apparent when account is taken of the fact that "achievement" is an ambiguous term and may be applied to a conduct which is most different from that of working.

The English language knows of two nouns (but only of one verb): play and game. The latter designates a playing activity subject to certain predetermined rules. One part plays against the other in a foot ball game or also in a game of chess. The winner experiences a sentiment of triumph, he also feels that he has achieved something (achieving victory is a English idiom) and is praised for his deeds.[6] But this

6 Whatever the educative significance of sportive activities may be, they are certainly not to he viewed as a preparation for work. Nor should one over-

achievement is not creative of values which would last, be it however, briefly, longer than the playing activity; society does not derive any "profit" from this achievement, at least, not directly for the relation of an Olympic victory to the Pindaric ode that celebrates it or to the statue which commemorates the victor is but that of an occasion. The prototype of this kind of achievement is the "record," But the reality of the human condition, the state of a community or of mankind is in no way influenced by the fact that someone arrived at a goal 36 seconds faster than another man. This means for mankind and in history as little as the fact that horse A was "beaten" by horse B at Longchamps.

In fact, however close play may come to work, there remains an essential difference which cannot he bridged. Play concerns exclusively the playing individual or individuals, it is socially irrelevant. Work, even when it is done only in the interest of the individual, is by its very nature related to society; the tool which a man creates for himself may be used also by an undetermined number of his fellows and the house he builds for himself will shelter others when the builder has passed away. Or to state in other terms what has been remarked above: all playing activity moves within the confines of subjectivity, whereas all working activity has consequences in the trans subjective world. Should a despot forbid playing golf and decree that all golf courses are to become public parks or terrain for building houses, nothing would be changed in the structure and the operations of society. But the disappearance of some working activity has consequences which affect the structure and the life of a whole society. The changes wrought by the Industrial Revolution, the technological progress and the ever expanding industrialization are as much the result of these positive factors as of the disappearance of the artisan and his kind of work.

The social relevance of work, as set over against the lack of such a relevance in play, constitutes a further profound difference between the two activities. Only in working man is fully responsible; playing,

---

look the fact that only those people are exposed to the beneficial influence of athletic activities who take actually part in them, not however those who are only spectators, perhaps, merely on the television screen. Furthermore, there is no guarantee that these influences will become effective outside of the athletic field. A. man may acquire the habits of fair play or of teamwork there and not hesitate to cheat at the card table or to desert his team in real life, where competition appears as so much more important.

he may do more or less as he likes.[7] Not even in the case of "games" is he obliged to abide strictly by the rules because he may change them at any time, provided his play mates agree. This is true of the play of children as well as of that of adults. What difference did it make to society that whist was replaced by bridge and that the rules of the latter were changed from time to time?

Only under certain conditions may activities related to play but not essential to it function as a preparation for future work. Thus when girls learn to handle needle and thread when making clothes for their dolls, or boys acquire some ability in handling tools in constructing or repairing things.

One more differentiating feature ought to he pointed out.

In certain kinds of play the playing child experiences besides and above the pleasure of function that of achievement and this feature may, as has been pointed out, allow to view play as a preparation for work. Nevertheless, there is a difference. In the case of play the whole performance and the resulting pleasure remain within the confines of subjectivity; even building some model of a machine has no significance for reality, that is, for communal life. However "true to life" the thing may look, it is but a copy and usually one on a notably reduced scale. It lacks the reference to society all work entails. It is very probable that this factor differentiates not only the work achieved but also the subjective experience.

Awareness of the relation to society does not mean exclusively development of the attitude of competition, although the opinion seems rather general to day that the awakening of the competitive spirit is a primary task of education. One may agree with this opinion – to a certain extent. We live to day indeed, in a highly competitive (and acquisitive) society. But a one-sided emphasis on competition is not without dangers; it may stimulate the learning activity of the child, but also inhibit it through discouragement.

There is, however, another tendency at work in every normal and healthy child: his curiosity and, correspondingly, the attraction everything exercises that is new. Aritsotle's famous dictum that "all men by nature want to know," applies to the child as well as to the adult

7 Sometimes, of course, playing may have trans subjective consequences. Children, for instance, may cause serious damages. But these consequences are purely accidental and have nothing to do with the essence of the playing activity.

(sometimes even more to the former than to the latter). It might well be that the child's interest in his scholastic activities will be more easily aroused, if he is told that he is entering a new field of experience, than when work is presented to him as another form of play. Some children seem to feel this way. A highly intelligent girl, who was sent to a very famous and expensive private school, asked her mother, after two weeks, whether she could not go to another school; no, she said, the children are very nice, the teachers also, everything was all right, but: "We play all the time, and I have as yet learned nothing."

During the first years in elementary school the child, of course, cannot be expected to appreciate the societal significance of work, as little as he is impressed by the old adage: *non scholae sed vitae discimus*. Life, being grown up, filling a place in society and similar ideas mean nothing to a child; he knows, indeed, that he will grow up; but he has but a faint idea of what this means.[8] One cannot expect either that the child will have an adequate understanding of such ideas as "social significance." But a competent teacher will be able to make the child see that he is entering a new phase of his life, setting out, as it were, on a voyage of discovery of a hitherto unknown land, acquiring a new status in reality, similar to, though not identical with, that of his parents and elders. This awakening of a new consciousness, of the realization that work does no longer allow for the arbitrariness of play but requires recognition of and submission to objective rules can, of course, take place only gradually. One cannot address a class of seven year old children as one might a class of students at a university. One may, however, rely on the child's interest in what is new and on the pleasure he finds in achievement.

Normal children will with but a little encouragement or, at least, when discouragement is carefully avoided, realize what it means "to work." They will be the first to acknowledge that our forefathers were right when they maintained that "there is a time for work and a time for play."

8 Further remarks on the child's relation to time may be found in the author's *Psicologia e Pedagogia del carattere*, a cura di R. Titone, Torino, 1961, Soc. Editrice Internazionale.

The legendary image of Freud
as a persecuted genius who finally attained
the fame he deserved in spite of hostile powers
is entirely without foundation.

THE FREUD LEGEND

Freud is known to his followers as well as to his critics as the one who first developed a psychological interpretation of neurotic syndromes and derived a method of treatment; as the one who expanded his conception of neurosis into a general theory of the human mind, and then made use of his principles for an explanation of the history of civilization and a critique of social and cultural phenomena. Thus, Freud's life work culminated in an encompassing theory of human nature, in what today is often referred to as a "philosophical anthropology."

Freud's ideas at first met severe criticism, were rejected and sometimes ridiculed. Gradually, however, they won recognition and, by virtue of their application to all sides of human life, achieved decisive influence far beyond the scope of psychiatry or psychology. Literature, cultural anthropology, education, sociology made extensive use of Freud's doctrine.

Great though Freud's success was, it never silenced criticism completely. Nor did his ideas remain unchanged. Not only did Freud himself repeatedly modify his theories, sometimes disconcerting thereby his most faithful disciples, but many of his notions were reinterpreted, so much so that often only the names were all that remained of the originals.[1]

All this is history. The many volumes of Freud's works, the immense number of publications elaborating on his ideas or also criticizing them, are there as reliable evidence. This history deals with Freud's work and has nothing to say either on the circumstances of his life and career or on his personality and its characteristic traits.

---

1 See, e.g., L. Salzman and I. H. Masserman, ed., *Modern Concepts of Psychoanalysis* (New York: Philosophical Library, 1962).

But there is, of course, a natural interest in the biography and in the person of a great man, whether he be a scientist, a creator of works of art, a statesman, a reformer, or a leader in any other field.

Freud himself published a short autobiography which, however, does not suffice for a complete and satisfactory picture. But there exist several shorter and longer biographies; the last and allegedly "definitive" one is that by Ernest Jones,[2] who through many years was not only a faithful, though sometimes critical, disciple, but a true friend. It was Dr. Jones who made it possible for Freud to leave Vienna, then ruled by the Nazis, and find an asylum in England.

In these biographies Freud appears as the persecuted genius who finally attained the lame he deserved in spite of all efforts on the part of hostile powers to prevent his victory. Envy and jealousy, one hears, did their best to handicap Freud's career. The faculty of the School of Medicine and the University as a whole, the Department of Education (*Ministeriuna für Unterricht*) are said to have denied to Freud the furtherance and promotion to which he was entitled. Most of all it was the anti-semitic sentiment allegedly dictating the policies of the University and the Government which became an insurmountable obstacle and brought it about that Freud became more famous and found far greater appreciation, and that the importance of his discoveries and ideas was recognized abroad more than in his own country. In fact, Freud himself once remarked that his renown "begins beyond the Austrian frontier."

This is the legend. It is a legend because there are no facts to support it.

This legendary picture had always appeared as highly questionable to those who knew Austria prior to 1918 – and for several years after the end of the war – and who were acquainted with the rules governing the procedures in academic affairs.

There were, however, no objective data available which might serve for a further development of this attitude of doubt, whereas the biographers of Freud presented their views with the assurance of men who feel that they are in possession of ascertained facts. The picture they drew is nevertheless pure legend. The question of how this legend came to be will be taken up later.

---

2 Ernest Jones, *The Life and Work of Sigmund Freud*, 3 vols. (New York: Basic Books, 1953-1956).

First it must be shown that the objective data are completely at variance with the legend. This has been rendered possible by the publication of a work in which all documents related to Freud's academic career are reproduced verbatim. These documents were, prior to the appearance of this work, quite unknown and also inaccessible.

Professor Joseph and Mrs. Renée Gicklhorn are the authors of a work on Freud's academic career, published in 1960.[3] Professor Gicklhorn, who died in 1957, taught History of Science at the University of Vienna. He and his wife started as botanists – she is at present a member of the staff of the Institute for Plant Physiology at the University of Vienna – and were led by their studies on the works of Austrian explorers and botanists to specialize in the history of science.

Mrs. Gicklhorn assembled all the pertinent documents, a task which required the examination of many thousands of reports, minutes of sessions or applications. After the premature decease of her husband, she had also to edit the documents and to add some further comments, whereas the sixty pages of the "Introduction and Interpretation" apparently are largely the work of the professor.

The authors emphasize that their purpose is exclusively to make available the hitherto missing objective evidence for a methodologically faultless history of Freud's relations with the School of Medicine and, at the same time, "to refute the truly monstrous reproaches and allegations which aim at discrediting the fame of Vienna and her cultural institutions and propagate false reports on the procedures of the University?" They point out that they are in no way concerned with Freud's doctrine, nor with his personality or his family life. Their intention is only to furnish the indispensable and reliable data for a future biography and to explain the significance of the several documents to readers who are neither acquainted with the legal and procedural rules which determined the actions of the faculty and the government nor possess an adequate knowledge of the general cultural climate that existed in Vienna prior to 1918 and for many years alter the end of the first world war and the dismemberment of the monarchy.

Confronted with the objectively ascertained facts, the Freud legend falls to pieces. Not one of its statements proves tenable. If a brute fact is presented correctly, its significance is thoroughly misunderstood.

3 Joseph & Renée Gicklhorn: *Sigmund Freuds akademische Laufbahn im Lichte der Dokumente* (Wien-Innsbruck: Verlag Urban & Schwarzenberg, 1960).

For instance, after his return from France, Freud joined the staff of a private institution for the treatment of children. It was not a hospital; only out patients were examined and treated. He hoped for and requested the permission of the Medical Faculty to be allowed to hold classes there on neurology. When his request was refused, he saw it as an expression of malevolence on the part of the Medical School. He disregarded, or never knew, the existence of a law which expressly forbade that classes be held in places not directly controlled by the School of Medicine. Again, he complained about the hostility of the faculty and the Department of Education because he could not obtain the promotion to the rank of an Associate Professor (*Extraordinarius*). In this case, too, he either did not know or disregarded the rules adopted by the Government and the Faculty, according to which an associate professor was supposed to be able to substitute for or to succeed the full professor lecturing on a recognized subject, particular stress being laid on teaching experience.

But Freud had applied for and received the right to teach neurology, which was not a recognized subject since it was linked up with psychiatry. This fact alone disqualified Freud, who, moreover, had but little interest in teaching. Again, Freud saw in the delay of his promotion and his finally receiving only the title but not the rank of an associate professor a manifestation of hostility on the part of the authorities.

Such details, of which many more could be mentioned, are important because all biographers have hitherto used as their only source the statements of Freud himself which they, moreover, misunderstood, for none of these authors had any direct knowledge of academic procedures, none cared to cheek the truth of the information thus obtained, and Dr. Jones, a foreigner, had but very vague, often quite mistaken ideas of the situation in Vienna.

It must be emphasized that all these men were perfectly bona fide: they saw no reason to doubt Freud's words.[4] And Freud himself was

---

4 One of the oldest followers of Freud, after having formulated a certain proposition, declared: "To the question, why I hold this thesis to be true, I shall reply, because Freud said so." It is understandable that such an unconditional belief in the *verba magistri*, spread, so to speak, from the statements on the doctrine to any utterance whatsoever. This may well have been one reason for the biographers to consider Freud's remarks on his personal life as a sufficient source and all further inquiry as superfluous. But there were other reasons, too.

no less bona fide: evidently he was convinced that things had happened as they appeared to him, often in retrospect. On neither side was there any trace of insincerity. But Freud's memory was not very reliable where his personal life and, especially, his unrealized expectations were concerned. Moreover, he harbored certain deeply ingrained preconceived ideas of whose truth he was so much convinced that he considered critical examination unnecessary.

The defectiveness of Freud's memory and the replacement of forgotten facts by the creations of his biased imagination resulted in his reports on past events sometimes being completely at variance with the documentary evidence. One striking example is the history of the grant which enabled Freud to pass several months at Paris and to work at the clinic of Charcot. According to Jones, this grant was made by the School of Medicine, arid Jones had no other source of information but the stories told by Freud. In fact, the grant was awarded by the government on the recommendation not of the Faculty but of the Academic Senate. Furthermore, the money was not destined exclusively for physicians, but was available alternatively to scholars belonging to the several schools of the University. Thirdly, the charter stated that the grant was to enable the recipient to study and work at an Austrian or German university; it was an exception in favor of Freud that he was allowed to go to Paris. Freud knew, of course, that one half of the stipend was to be given before the recipient left and the second half after his return. But it was several months before the second payment was made. Freud in his later years saw therein one more proof of ill will and hostility on the part of the authorities. He had forgotten that this payment was dependent on the presentation of a report on his activities during his absence. And it was he who caused the delay because he submitted this report only several months after his return (Document 15; the first page of Freud's report is reproduced in fig. 7).

This is but one instance of several in which Freud made responsible for certain more or less unpleasant experiences the hostile forces which be believed to he at work, whereas in point of fact these events were of Freud's own doing. But it would take up too much space to recount all the discrepancies between the objective facts on the one hand, and the statements of Freud and his biographers on the other.

The statements of Freud's biographers suffer from three serious defects: (1) absolute and exclusive reliance on Freud's statements, (2) ignorance of the rules and procedures of universities – none of the biographers had any personal knowledge of these matters – or even, in the case of Dr. Jones, of the situation in Austria during the reign of Franz Joseph I and the first ten years or so of the Republic, (3) complete lack of knowledge of even a minimum of historiographic methodology. Under these circumstances it becomes understandable that the authors of the several biographies have drawn a distorted picture of their hero and his career.

Here is one instance: When Dr. Jones congratulated Freud on receiving the title of full professor (*ordinarius*), Freud remarked: "It is only a title." Freud, of course, knew very well that he could not attain the position of a full professor, since such positions were held only by the heads of clinics or institutes and neither the Faculty nor the Government could create a new professorship. Hence, his words were meant as an explanation to prevent a misunderstanding on Dr. Jones's part. But because the latter did not know anything about such matters, he misunderstood Freud's words as if Freud had said: "I have been given the title, although I ought to have been made a full professor." And Dr. Jones saw therein a further indication of lasting hostility on the part of the authorities.

On this occasion the fault was wholly that of the biographer. Generally, however, it was Freud himself who saw everywhere manifestations of malevolence. He knew, in fact, only three reasons for anyone not to recognize the truth of his ideas and the greatness of their discoverer. First, the natural reluctance ("resistance") of a person still dominated by his "unconscious" and tyrannized by his "super ego," and whose ego was, as Freud once put it, "not master in his own house." Analysis would enable such a person to realize the interplay of drives, the lasting effects of early experiences, the "symbolic" nature of his character traits, and so on, and thus recognize the basic truths concerning human nature as revealed by psychoanalysis.[5]

5 Because Freud was convinced that without the self-knowledge which psychoanalysis alone could supply no one could free himself of the tyranny mentioned above and therefore recognize the causes of neurotic troubles, he made it a requirement for any one desirous of being a psychoanalyst that he be first of all analyzed himself. For one or another reason he made, at least, one exception. Professor Paul Schilder, perhaps the most gifted of Freud's followers, told me that he had not been analyzed and never intended to be. He was an Assistant of Wagner von Jauregg, and later the

This was an excusable reason for antagonism which could be remedied if the critic agreed to let himself be analyzed. But, according to Freud, there was a second reason which made people reject the new doctrine because by doing so they aimed at Freud himself as a person. These enemies, he believed, were prompted by envy, by malevolence, by the fear that their traditional views would be discredited. The book by the Gicklhorns shows clearly that Freud thoroughly misinterpreted the situation. Nowhere in the minutes of the Faculty, in the reports of its committees or in the correspondence with the Government does one find the slightest trace of enmity. Quite the contrary, there was a marked tendency to further Freud, and his failure to obtain what he wanted was not the result of malevolence but of his being unaware of the prevailing conditions and the legal situation.

The third and, in Freud's view, the most powerful reason was anti-semitism. Dr. and Mrs. Gickihorn have carried out their painstaking research not only for the sake of furnishing an objective report on Freud's academic career, but also to straighten out the warped picture which many people harbor of Austria and Austrian mentality of sixty and even of thirty five years ago. This picture is, as the authors point out, the effect of a reading back into the past features which came to the fore mainly through the influence of German racism since 1933. The authors keep strictly within the boundaries which they had set for their work. They say nothing of Freud's doctrine and the reaction it released or of his personality. But to understand Freud's incessantly repeated denunciation of anti-semitism as the chief source of all the obstacles he encountered, or claimed to have encountered, a short digression dealing with his personality appears indispensable.

In one of the conversations I had with an outstanding psychoanalyst of Washington, D.C., recently deceased, I referred to the astonishing achievement of Freud's self analysis. The analyst agreed but added that Freud was never able to discover the sources of certain of his traits, that he, perhaps, was not even aware of their existence, especially of his marked aggressivity and his extreme intolerance. For the latter term one may substitute that of a rigid authoritarianism which perhaps describes Freud's conduct even better.

---

head of the psychiatric ward at Bellevue Hospital, New York, and was killed in a traffic accident in 1939.

Early in his career he had a violent conflict with the head of the ward in the General Hospital to which he was attached. As a consequence Dr. Scholz forbade him to present patients in his courses on nervous diseases. He broke with Dr. Breuer, to whom he was indebted in several respects. The history of one of Breuer's patients – later published as the first of the *Studies on Hysteria* by Joseph Breuer and Sigmund Freud, Vienna, 1895 – aroused Freud's interest in the psychology of neurotic troubles, even before he left for Paris. The chapter on the theory of neurosis – or, as the authors said then, of "hysteria" – stemmed from Breuer and is expressly so designated. Breuer furthered his younger colleague as best he could and also helped him out by a substantial loan when Freud's income was still insufficient. It may well be that these obligations were felt by Freud as intolerable for in him the need to be independent and to rule seems to have been very strong.

He likewise broke with Fliess, after years of friendship and extensive correspondence.[6]

The traits previously referred to, however, become most evident in Freud's dealings with his followers. He defined certain basic propositions which everyone had to accept who wanted to become or to remain a member of the Psychoanalytic Association. Whenever he came to the conclusion that one of these propositions had to be abandoned or modified, he demanded that the new doctrine be adopted without questioning. He was, of course, willing to discuss these points, to explain them, but the decision was to be ultimately his and his alone. If anyone refused to follow him, he was in the literal sense of the term "excommunicated." And Freud not only dropped all relations with these people but spoke of them in a contemptuous and most harsh manner. Freud was convinced that the "dissenters" had learned from him all they had to say. Accordingly, he saw in them not only men who had strayed from the path of truth, but who also gave proof of a shocking ingratitude.

6 Apparently the only person who was able to remain on good terms with Freud in spite of some rather deep differences was Ludwig Binswanger. Why this was so cannot be ascertained. Perhaps the reason was that the two men had more in common than their interest in psychoanalysis. Like Freud, Binswanger was a man of universal culture, whereas the other disciples hardly transcended the boundaries of psychoanalysis even when they wrote on art, literature or other aspects of civilization.

The attitude which Freud assumed in regard to Alfred Adler, C. G. Jung, O. Rank or W. Stekel is sufficiently known, so that examples become superfluous. It must, however, be emphasized that Freud here, too, acted *optima fide.*

It is not within the scope of this article to attempt a characterization of Freud's highly complicated personality. This is, probably, not yet feasible; one will have to wait until further data, for example, objectively presented letters, will be at our disposal. But the few remarks here submitted seem necessary because they may furnish the key to Freud's unfounded and tenaciously repeated statements.

Aggressivity and authoritarianism, of which one is unaware, together with the consciousness of originality and superiority, lead easily to attributing motives of hostility to everyone who really or supposedly becomes an obstacle. One can understand that Freud saw in the difficulties he encountered manifestations of ill will or envy. It is much less easy to understand why be was obsessed – the word is not too strong – by the idea that he was a victim of anti-semitism.

Neither in the action of the faculty nor in those of the government can one discover any indication of an antisemitic sentiment. In the former there were always some full professors (*ordinarii*), heads of clinics or institutes, who were Jews. The same is true of the School of Arts and Sciences (Philosophical Faculty). The Emperor Francis Joseph had certainly no predilection for Jews; but he was an eminently just man unwilling to discriminate among his subjects[7] – for example, he named the famous Grecist and historian of Greek philosophy, Theodor Gomperz, a member of the Upper House, knighted the Jewish actor Sonnenthal, consented to the election of a Jewish convert as Archbishop of Olmütz; another convert became canon and main preacher at the Cathedral of St. Stephen.

Francis Joseph disapproved of anti-semitism, first, because he was a good Catholic, secondly, because he saw in this trend a disruptive force. This became evident when the Christian Social majority of the Viennese Municipal Council elected Dr. Karl Lueger[8] as Mayor. The Mayor of Vienna had to be confirmed in his position by the Emperor,

7 The Austrian Penal Law provided the same protection against defamation of the Protestant (Lutheran and Calvinistic) and the Hebrew faith as of that of the Catholic Church.

8 Pronounced Loo-éhger.

who refused twice to sign the decree and gave in, reluctantly, only the third time.

Anti-semitism was one of the points in the political program of the Christian Socialists, which was mainly the party of the lower middle class. Accordingly, it was mostly a question of economic competition, religious elements playing a very minor role and racism none at all. Only a small but vociferous party of extreme German Nationalists professed a violent racial antagonism. Its leader was the Representative von Schoenerer, many of whose ideas Hitler took over.

The anti-semitism of the Lueger era was far less aggressive than that of later times; it was also less consistent. Dr. Lueger used to have weekly card parties in a certain coffee house, and one of the group was a Jew. One day some prominent Christian Socialists pointed out to Lueger that it was not right of him to admit a Jew to his company. Whereupon Dr. Lueger hit the desk with the flat of his hand, exclaiming: "Who is and who is not a Jew, that's for me to decide!" This was, in fact, a widely spread sentiment, although other people would hardly have expressed it in the same manner. They spoke, indeed, of "the Jews" as of a danger, as possessing all sorts of undesirable qualities, made them responsible for many, especially economic, mishaps; but almost everyone would make an exception for this or that individual Jew he knew.

This kind of anti-semitism could not have influenced Freud's academic career, for the reasons mentioned above. The idea of an anti-semitic conspiracy, if one may call it so, originated in the mind of Freud, was propagated by incompetent biographers and popularizers and believed by the large number of those who did not know anything of the actual state of affairs in old Austria. This ignorance made it possible for the picture which Austria presented in the last years before the German invasion to be projected back into the past, as if it had always existed.

Freud was blind to all facts which were not in accord with his preconceived ideas and, therefore, did not become aware of certain quite obvious contradictions in his own statements. On the one hand, for instance, he made anti-semitism responsible for the rejection of his ideas, on the other he found fault with the medical circles in Vienna because he met unbelief and criticism there. But he overlooked the fact that a large number of physicians in Vienna were Jews and not less opposed to his doctrine than their gentile colleagues. He accused the Faculty and the Government because he could not obtain what he desired, but did not realize that his demands could not be fulfilled owing to legal reasons.

People believed him because of the unfortunately common habit of crediting authority on all sorts of questions to one who is an authority in a special field. This tendency was, of course, particularly strong among his admirers. In this way the Freud legend developed and was taken for historical truth, although it appeared improbable to some even before the publication of the documents. But since we now possess, thanks to the work of Dr. and Mrs. Gicklhorn, the means to reconstruct the historical facts, the legend has lost all credibility.[9]

The history of the psychoanalytic movement must be rewritten. The picture of Freud's personality as drawn by his biographers must be subjected to a new and searching inquiry. Certain details in the existing biographies, especially in that of Dr. Jones, have already taken on a new significance; possibly one may foresee the direction these new studies will have to take.[10] But such matters fall outside the scope of this report.

9 The authors have made their discoveries available to the American Freud Archives. They note that in recent years the references to the "anti-semitic conspiracy" have become much less frequent.

10 One may find some remarks on the place of Freud's work in the history of ideas in the first of my four lectures on *Existentialism and Psychiatry* (Springfield, Ill., 1961).

INDEX